Praise for *Chakras, th*

"An excellent book tying to standing of trauma. Truly unique in her approach, the author writes with great compassion and well-articulated science as she explores the various ways the vagus nerve plays out in each chakra. With many easy-to-follow exercises for healing and awakening, I highly recommend this book."

—**ANODEA JUDITH**, PhD, author of *Wheels of Life*, *Chakra Yoga*, and *Eastern Body, Western Mind*

"You are all equipped with a highly intelligent vehicle that carries you through life: your body. C. J. Llewelyn has given you the user's manual to help you maintain and optimize the complex intersection of your nervous and endocrine systems that form the physiological basis of your energetic body and the chakras. The vagus nerve, also known as the wandering nerve, is a mind-body superhighway of communication. The practices within this book are the keys that help you to successfully navigate stress while allowing you to find greater freedom in your body and mind."

—**ARIELLE SCHWARTZ**, PhD, psychologist and author of *Applied Polyvagal Theory in Yoga*

About the Author

C. J. Llewelyn, MEd, LPC, is a licensed professional counselor and marriage and family therapist. Her passion is combining the psychological, physical, and spiritual to heal trauma and facilitate personal and spiritual growth in her clients. C. J. is a trained Internal Family Systems Therapist and is certified in EMDR (Eye Movement Desensitization Reprocessing). She utilizes polyvagal theory, energy psychology, and a knowledge of the chakras and subtle energies in her work. She is also a reiki master in the lineage of Dr. Mikao Usui and and a faculty member of the Shift Network. Visit her at CJLlewelyn.com.

CHAKRAS
THE VAGUS
NERVE AND YOUR
SOUL

CHAKRAS
THE VAGUS
NERVE AND YOUR
SOUL

JOURNEYING TO WELLNESS THROUGH SUBTLE ENERGY AND YOUR NERVOUS SYSTEM

C. J. LLEWELYN, MED, LPC

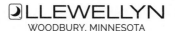
LLEWELLYN
WOODBURY, MINNESOTA

FIRST EDITION
First Printing, 2025

Book design by Christine Ha
Cover design by Shannon McKuhen
Interior illustrations
    Figures 1, 2, 4–11 by the Llewellyn Art Department
    Figure 3
        The brain, in right profile with the glossopharyngeal and vagus nerves and, to the right, a view of the base of the brain. Photolithograph from 1940 after a 1543 woodcut. Source: Wellcome Collection.

Llewellyn Publications is a registered trademark of Llewellyn Worldwide Ltd.

Library of Congress Cataloging-in-Publication Data
Names: Llewelyn, C. J., author.
Title: Chakras, the vagus nerve, and your soul : journeying to wellness
  through subtle energy and your nervous system / C. J. Llewelyn, MEd,
  LPC.
Description: First edition. | Woodbury, MN : Llewellyn Publications, a
  division of Llewellyn Worldwide Ltd., [2025] | Includes bibliographical
  references. | Summary: "The chakras and vagus nerve are mirrors of each
  other; learning to tune into what they are telling you is vital. With
  more than forty-five exercises to enhance your learning, this book
  teaches you to trust your inner wisdom"-- Provided by publisher.
Identifiers: LCCN 2024055701 (print) | LCCN 2024055702 (ebook) | ISBN
  9780738779393 (paperback) | ISBN 9780738779485 (ebook)
Subjects: LCSH: Chakras--Psychological aspects. | Chakras--Health aspects.
  | Vagus nerve. | Healing--Psychological aspects.
Classification: LCC BF1442.C53 .L544 2025 (print) | LCC BF1442.C53
  (ebook) | DDC 294.5/43--dc23/eng/20250106
LC record available at https://lccn.loc.gov/2024055701
LC ebook record available at https://lccn.loc.gov/2024055702

Llewellyn Publications
A Division of Llewellyn Worldwide Ltd.
2143 Wooddale Drive
Woodbury, MN 55125-2989
www.llewellyn.com

Printed in the United States of America

Other Books by C. J. Llewelyn

Chakras and the Vagus Nerve

Disclaimer

The material in this book is not intended as a substitute for trained medical or psychological advice. Readers are advised to consult their personal healthcare professionals regarding treatment. The publisher and the author assume no liability for any injuries caused to the reader that may result from the reader's use of the content contained herein and recommend common sense when contemplating the practices described in the work. The publisher and author also endorse seeking a qualified, licensed trauma-informed therapist if you are in need, as this book is not a substitute for trauma-related psychotherapy.

CONTENTS

———•————•———

EXERCISES

Chapter 6

Chapter 7

Chapter 8

Chapter 9

Chapter 10

FIGURES

───•───•───

LETTER TO THE READER

Dear Weary Traveler,

How's the life journey going? Have you had some pitfalls, brilliant moments, joys, hard climbs, and restful stops as you have walked your path? Or are you clinging to the mile markers each time you drag your feet to the next fork in the road? Have the people you've encountered been kind or rough? How have you treated those you have met? Do you join with people in fear or laughter? Kindness or brutality? Have you followed some who have led you through dark forests or wide-open roads? Have you chosen your mentors wisely or rejected all help? The mundane stretches of the journey instill some doubt about why you're even doing this, don't they? Ugh, that doubt. Double ugh about the mundane. Makes you just want to look for diversions, doesn't it?

Along the way, have you listened to your internal compass to help you know where you are going? Did you even know you were equipped with one? Where is it, you ask? Well, it's everywhere within you, and its life force reaches outside of you. This compass has steered your ancestors out of millions of years of adversity, pain, and sorrow. It has drawn them toward love and acceptance and compelled them to thrive as they have journeyed this earth plane. Just like it does for you. Just like it does for all of us. This compass is your nervous system, specifically your vagus nerve.

That intricate nerve detects danger and safety—real or imagined—along your way. And just like the energy in a lodestone that fuels a compass needle to point to the earth's poles, the cosmic frequency in your body fuels your vagus nerve. Many call this frequency Soul. Amazingly, this life force drives all parts of your body, as Soul needs it for the discovery mission it's on. Your Soul is compelling, astonishing, and curious about this journey you chose. Yet, while Soul, in its infinite energy and wisdom, is up for the expedition, sometimes the body tires. When this happens, your human mind, with its imperfect interpretation of the cosmos, grows doubtful with limiting beliefs.

So, slow down, be gentle with yourself, and listen differently.

You can hear the lure of your Soul through the elaborate fibers of the vagus nerve. If you attune, the messages of the vagus echo along the body and radiate outward from fibrous centers that ancient Hindu yogis called the chakras, or cakras.[1]

I offer to you, dear traveler, a way to honor the dichotomous nature of your earthly existence and your spirituality. Allow for grace and sustenance to your physical well-being. Reach for gratitude. Rest along the way. This will serve your Soul's journey well. Taking care of your physical form—including that beautiful vagus nerve—serves a Soulful intention that you might not immediately discern. Trust that you are on the path you need to be and that you can turn to this compass in your most confusing times.

With blessings and compassion,
C. J. Llewelyn, MEd, LPC

---

1. Avalon, *The Serpent Power*, 103.

INTRODUCTION

I want you to consider this book, *Chakras, the Vagus Nerve, and Your Soul: Journeying to Wellness Through Subtle Energy and Your Nervous System,* a travel guide. This guide comes with operating instructions because no journey that you embark on can happen unless you efficiently steer and care for the vehicle that takes you where you need to go. In this case, the vehicle is your body. Its navigational system is the vagus nerve. The sensors that bounce light off of your vehicle on to others are your chakras.

Befriend and care for this vehicle because the energy that fuels it is your Soul. Your Soul communicates along the vagal nerve fibers. It flows to the nerve plexuses, where the energy condenses and expresses outside your body. The ancients called this energy the cakras, or chakras. It is symbiotic. It directs out like a beacon, then dispatches inward, up along the vagus nerve and all that this nerve connects to. Like the sensors in a self-driving vehicle, it tells you when to slow down or speed up, not get too close, or not hit a curb.

This sensory system is not perfect. Like the wiring in a car when it is not maintained, it can misinterpret signals. This is particularly the case when you have experienced trauma. Your wiring is intended to store data, to avoid further crashes. If you have had several crashes, your system might interpret everything as a potential accident waiting to happen. It can also stop working altogether and not read any dangers in front of you.

Trauma

So you can understand how to avoid misfires in your vehicle, let's first clarify what trauma is. *Trauma* is a word that gets tossed around a lot these days. In many ways, this is a good thing. It means the world is developing an understanding of how harsh experiences affect us. It gives people definitions so they can understand what has happened to them and learn how to effectively get help. However, like any term that gets overused, it can lose its true meaning and get watered down.

Trauma is a psychological and emotional response to an event or a series of events that are deeply distressing or disturbing. These are abruptions; they jolt you out of a place of physical or emotional safety. Traumatic events can be childhood or spousal abuse, accidents, natural disasters, loss, or any other situation that threatens your sense of security.[2] These events can overwhelm your ability to cope with further stressors. A person who has experienced traumatic events can feel helpless or weakened. Trauma leaves you with an inability to connect Soulfully because you interpret the heightened physiological reactions in your body as emotions. This can make you afraid to feel because you believe feeling always hurts.

When trauma is unresolved, it has long-lasting effects. Your nervous system—your vehicle's wiring—will either be on high alert or shut you down to conserve energy. Your body misinterprets the moment. Your wiring struggles to read if you are safe in this situation because it *feels* like past situations. This happens because the trauma hasn't been fully processed by your nervous system. The traumatic situations are not being stored as past events. Your body remains active, and you respond as if the events

---

2. Friedman, Keane, and Resick, *Handbook of PTSD*, 230.

are still occurring. This looks like flashbacks, intrusive thoughts, or intense emotional (physiological) reactions.

Trauma responses don't always reveal themselves in forceful ways. Like that undetectable rattle in the engine of your car, you can feel regularly annoyed or edgy, moody, overwhelmed, or shutdown. Your mind struggles to focus. Trauma steals time. When your body feels trapped in the past, it cannot move forward on its journey. You stay put because the world feels distressing. Desires feel unattainable. Venturing out feels scary or at the very least exhausting. This overwhelm keeps you from fully embarking upon your spiritual expedition.

This book is intended to inform you and offer supportive resources, not clear the trauma from your system. Keeping with the car metaphor, there is a difference between a collision specialist and a mechanic. If any of these trauma descriptions look familiar, seek out the work of an informed, licensed trauma therapist in the mental health field that is trained in neuro-experiential modalities (i.e., Brainspotting, Internal Family Systems, or Eye Movement Desensitization Reprocessing). You will get a good diagnostic assessment and a plan to repair. This is the mechanic your engine needs.

Approaching and healing the emotional body is by no means an exact science because we humans, how we interpret life experiences, and how we store our pain, is expressively unique. However, we do have modalities and theoretical frameworks (like the ones I just mentioned) that have been studied for decades. These are changing the paradigm of healing. The polyvagal theory, developed by Dr. Stephen Porges in 1994, is one of those.[3]

Polyvagal theory explains how the autonomic nervous system, the vagus nerve, influences your emotional regulation and stress

---

3. Porges, *Polyvagal Theory.*

responses. It highlights the importance of safety as the fundamental key to what drives you. Polyvagal theory conceives the three branches of the vagus nerve—ventral vagal, sympathetic, and dorsal vagal complex—work in unison to keep your body responsive to dangers. Simply put, you cannot access your spiritual state unless your body feels safe.

Your vagus nerve is the largest autonomic nerve in your body. It is cranial nerve X that extends from the medulla oblongata, which is at the base of your skull. This massive nerve keeps your heart pumping, your lungs breathing, and your food digesting as you go about your day. This cranial nerve communicates with other nerve fibers in your eyes, middle ear, and facial muscles. It stimulates your swallowing and digestion. When you experience medical issues, such as heart, stomach, intestine, liver, kidney, respiratory, or throat issues, you are more than likely also struggling with the health of your autonomic nervous system, as the vagus innervates these and other organs. What this nerve also does is keep you safe.

The vagus receives and imprints life experiences onto your neural circuitry. So, when there is another similar occurrence, your system can respond. Sometimes the amazing intelligence of this nerve, along with the interpretations from the brain, may do too good of a job. Your system may interpret a past traumatic episode as a present-day one. When this happens, you may freeze into submission, get combative, or not be able to be present to the moment.

Polyvagal theory put into words what trauma therapists saw for decades—that neurobiological responses to perceived threats are not over-the-top emotions. As I say in my workshops with other therapists, polyvagal theory helped us take the shame out of our clients' beliefs about themselves. When you can clear trauma and reestablish an accurate measure of safety in your body, many stress-related medical issues cease to be primary problems.[4] You can then connect to your inner world with greater ease. In this way, healing the psychological is a very spiritual act.

The Chakras

Chakras are energy centers that emanate from your body. They are described in various Hindu, Yogic, and Tantric traditions that (even thousands of years ago) suggested these energies are aligned with various nerve endings or plexus. While we have numerous energy centers in the body, I am focused on the seven main ones that align with the vagus nerve and connecting organs. As a trauma therapist and reiki master, I have seen how these energy centers align with the vagus and connecting nerves as they run along the torso, neck, and head. I have been intrigued by how the messages the ancients discerned within each chakra seem synonymous with the childhood issues stored in my clients' bodies. These messages don't necessarily have to be born of trauma. I have also noticed general patterns of how the dimensions of our everyday humanness present along this informational path. These energy centers perfectly reflect the human struggle.

I do not use any ancient Sanskrit terms as I discuss the chakras throughout this book. Learning about your autonomic nervous system and various methods of healing and attuning to your subtle energies is enough to ask of anyone. My clinical training urges me, instead, to break the chakras down into those dimensions of your psychological human experience. When they show up in sessions, they do not betray the ancients.

In the second chapter, you will find a schema of how I see this energy run along your autonomic nerve branches. Later in

---

4. Ogden and Fisher, *Sensorimotor Psychotherapy*.

the book, there will be another diagram of the chakras, and yes, there will be a figure of the vagus nerve. My description of the chakras and their dimensions runs from the bottom up. In trauma processing, working with the energy of the body and nervous system is proven to be the most permanent approach to healing.[5] So, it makes sense to begin the discussion with the chakras, nerves, and their connecting organs closest to the earth. Your body holds your first and deepest memories, emotional states, and wisdom because, as I posit, it is the temporary home of your Soul.

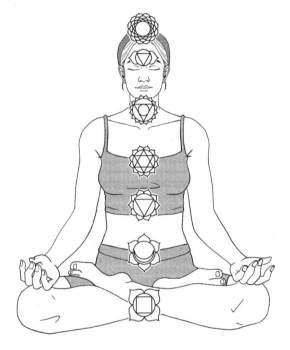

Figure 1: Chakras

---

5. Lanius, Paulsen, and Corrigan, *Neurobiology and Treatment of Traumatic Dissociation*, 457.

I call the chakras that run from your pelvis to your solar plexus region the essential chakras. Through the lens of human development these chakras reflect your life journey. They align with the subdiaphragmatic (below your respiratory diaphragm) processes that the vagus nerve automatically performs. They are digestive and anciently protective.

The first energy center is the root chakra. It holds the messages of survival. Without your physical self, your Soul cannot be here. Your body connects to the earth for its sustenance and connects to others for safety. Therefore, I call the root chakra the dimension of your body.

Your young body is highly dependent upon caregivers to stay alive. The patterns of how you connect to the people who raise you show up deeply in the sacral chakra. You feel both the loving connection and the lack of it in your belly. I call this energy center the dimension of emotion.

Once you develop some autonomy from caregivers, you form identities in the outside world. How you engage with others, how you position yourself within your community, and how you see yourself through the tasks you are asked to perform is shaped in the dimension of mind. Ego identities are felt strongly in the solar plexus chakra, especially if you struggle with how you identify within your world. These three chakras align with the very human processes of digestion, excretion, and reproduction. When you feel a lack of safety, you most certainly experience disruption in your organs connected to the vagus nerve in this part of your body. We all do.

The chakras above the diaphragm align with a branch of the vagus that manages your physiological calm and brings you to a place of connection with others. I call these the evolving chakras, since once you are able to maintain some equanimity, you can reach the deeper wisdom within yourself. This is one of the reasons so many people love the heart chakra. It is a powerful source of healing because the vagal branches connected to the heart and lungs are designed to slow you down and help you regroup. This is how you evolve in your ability to engage with yourself and others. This is where calm, reflection, connection, and intuitive awareness begin.

The throat chakra makes up a wonderful complexity of vagal fibers that not only allow you to speak but hear. This is the only energy center that manifests sound and, I think, is the most powerful of all the chakra centers for connection.

The third eye chakra, the dimension of spirituality, brings you to your inner world through symbolism and imagery. Ocular nerves in your middle brain region send signals to the vagus nerve. These nerves play a role in the experience of your internal, spiritual messages. They are also a vital component utilized in several modalities of trauma healing.[6] This energy center is also situated near the key ventricles of the brain.

The crown chakra, which I call the dimension of empathy, engages you in a bigger spiritual picture. It aligns with the ventricle system's cerebrospinal fluid and important glands that play a role in the stress response.[7] When you attune to this energy center on the front top of your skull, your system can flow more smoothly—all the way down to your root chakra. It is also the energy center that extends outward to a higher realm and acts like a homing device as you connect to Universal Source.

All of these chakras represent the whole of your felt experience as it works along your neurobiology. Staying attuned to your

---

6. Grand, *Brainspotting.*
7. Zappaterra, "Connection to Source via the Cerebrospinal Fluid."

felt experience is key to knowing what to tend to and what to heal in your life. This includes alleviating stored trauma responses that have imprinted in your body for years.

What to Expect from This Book

My first book, *Chakras and the Vagus Nerve: Tap Into the Healing Combination of Subtle Energy and Your Nervous System*, shared my observation of the alignment of the vagus nerve and chakras. That book covers a lot of what. This book, *Chakras, the Vagus Nerve, and Your Soul: Journeying to Wellness Through Subtle Energy and Your Nervous System*, presents more how. *How* to develop an awareness of what your embodied Soul is communicating. *How* to sort through the human communication systems versus the Soulful ones. *How* to move energy through your system. *How* to live a more balanced and peaceful life. *How* to build a healthy nervous system and lifestyle. There are a lot more exercises in this book. My aim is to offer a deeper map that assists you in creating a Soulfully human experience.

Just like the schema of a large map in a public area, we mark the beginning of the journey with the first section, "You Are Here." Chapter 1 breaks down how you disconnect from your Soulful, intuitive ways by approaching life with doubt. Chapter 2 covers the three states of the vagus nerve and how they work as your navigational system based on polyvagal theory. Chapter 3 brings you to the earthly experiences of the essential chakras as they align with the vagus. Chapter 4 introduces you to how heavenly experiences of the essential chakras and vagus nerve facilitate healing and lead you to deeper spiritual awareness.

Once you know your equipment for the trip, the second part, "The Way Forward," shows you how to use your gear by means of a mindful approach. Chapter 5 introduces mindful exercises and concepts to keep you present and safe. Chapter 6 breaks down some health-related issues to watch for along the way. Chapter 7 introduces you to ways to care for your vagus nerve, as it is your primary navigation device.

The third section, "The Journey on Your Terms," discusses how to pull this information together so you can live your best ride. Chapter 8 discusses the miraculous ways we heal when we can trust our inner messages and wisdom by going within. Chapter 9 breaks down how to listen to your vagal tone and discover how your nervous system is doing. Chapter 10 deepens the concept of mindfulness by how to approach life with acceptance so you can reach inner peace.

Halfway through writing this book, there became an unintended outcome for me. I was diagnosed with shingles for the first time in my life. Ironically, this happened while I was writing the chapter on vagus nerve health. Despite my best efforts of practicing what I preach, here I was, experiencing the physical and emotional results of what happens when stressors get too real and affect your nervous system. Very humbling. My book was no longer just a passionate project to send out into the world. It became a full-on experiential one.

The healer was suddenly in need of deep healing. So, deep I went. Deeper and deeper. I meditated in traditional Vipassana style each morning to still my thoughts and center my body. I brought back a regular yoga routine. I slowed my usual exercise style of cycling for miles and pushing myself too hard and engaged in more mindful walking. Walking my friend's dog, Winnie, became a nice way to coregulate with her and nature. I also listened to my Soul about what breath work and movement it wanted my body to do in order to reinstate healing. I tended not only to my body's messages but opened to an internal wisdom that guides us all. Reaching deep was profound and hopeful. My hope is that I can share these skill sets and information to help you.

Chakras, the Vagus Nerve, and Your Soul: Journeying to Wellness Through Subtle Energy and Your Nervous System is intended as a road map for hope and comfort. It is a thoughtful way to help you get some breathing room and regain the Soulful connection to yourself.

Safe travels.

PART 1
YOU ARE HERE

CHAPTER 1

BE THE CURIOUS TRAVELER

H ave you ever traveled to a new place? What was the first thing that struck you about it? Was it the feel of the weather on your skin? New scents in the air? New sounds? As you recall that memory, where do you feel it in your body now?

When you have wonderful new experiences, your senses are heightened. That's because your nervous system and brain undergo several changes in response to that newness. When you are on vacation, trying out a new restaurant, or attempting to learn a new language, your system reorganizes its communication connections. This allows you to easily retain new information. That newness is organized in your body as a felt experience.

New information brings on an adaptability in your brain and nervous system called neuroplasticity. It is like a flexible muscle, and with neuroplasticity your internal system can more easily adjust to changing experiences. How can you become more flexible in your way of being and experiencing things? Start by being curious.

Curiosity activates the brain region responsible for decision-making and problem-solving, which then manages emotions. Being curious helps you shift your thinking and behavior in response to new situations. It keeps you open to new ideas. Curiosity suspends judgment. It makes it easy to breathe into the unknown and allows you to be in the moment. You feel safe because you are in the moment.

You don't have to travel to exotic, faraway lands to have this very present, very open connection. You can be in the same old place that you have always been and bring on a brand-new experience. Just look at that old thing in a new way. See like you have never been in your living room before. Listen to your partner's very familiar voice in a different way. Pause. Notice one of your five senses with specific care. Breathe in. Pay attention to how your body relearns that moment. Return to that inquisitive feeling you had in childhood.

Just like that, you've pulled more flexibility into your nervous system.

Your brain is in child mode when you are curious. You're open and experimental and willing to explore, which means faltering isn't a problem. Because children examine things, they can be uncertain and still want to understand. When you stop being curious, you lose connection to yourself. You lose that childlike randomness and joy.

So, what is the opposite of curiosity? Perhaps anything that blocks your present awareness and keeps you in old patterns of thinking. Judgment, negativity, and cynicism block that inquisitive flow because you have approached something with a presupposition that the outcome won't be very nice or will be the same as it always is. Those negative beliefs keep your brain and nervous system locked in patterns of fear.

Fear Is Disconnect

Fear stimulates a defensive response. This reinforces a world view that supports self-protective measures, consciously and unconsciously.

That's because fear creates a different neurobiological pattern than curiosity does. When you are fearing, your system gets over- or under-stimulated.[8] Thinking drops down into the part of your brain that reacts. Then defensive posturing trickles into your life as a regular pattern. You come at relationships, work, and your own nature in mistrusting, doubtful ways.

When you are constantly on the lookout, you aren't accurately reading your body's signals. That's because fear is constantly organizing a powerful, coordinated response in the nervous system. Its only priority is survival. That can get confusing when you are in a place that is not scary and is supposed to be pleasant.

When the fear response is activated too frequently, you experience chronic stress. That stress can reduce your vagus nerve's ability to regulate all that it is in charge of. That means vagal tone—which is how adaptable your vagus nerve is to managing the system—lowers. You can struggle with heart, digestive, and respiratory issues. Inflammation can be a regular struggle. Hair and skin are affected. Your body wants you to listen to it during both the easiest and the hardest parts of your journey.

Part of listening to your body is to be curious about the signals it is sending.[9] Even in times of stress, you can inquire. Notice your heartbeat; take a breath. Be curious about the tension and where it is in your body. Take note of how your body is reacting. Did that response match the situation? How are you able to recover from that situation? What does your body need?

Your epic life journey might not be over mountains and into new countries. It might be about meeting the people who moved in next door or taking on a new job that provides a better life.

---

8. Panksepp and Biven, *The Archaeology of Mind*, 390.
9. LeDoux, *The Emotional Brain*, 23.

When you can stay present to how your body feels during those times, you have claimed your personal power. Being in the present moment is what helps you to understand your reality. Even if someone else tries to tell you differently, you will know what you need because you will be staying curious.

EXERCISE
Writing Prompt: Who's Got Your Power?

When you are facing a life experience that is upsetting but the person you are with is minimizing your feelings, this shows up in your body as an energy blockage. "It wasn't that big of a deal." "You're okay." "I don't know why this bothers you."

I'm sure you have heard these responses before. Did they make you doubt what happened? Did you start to think the person minimizing your experience was right and you were wrong? Having someone deny your reality surfaces as anxiety, tenseness, stomachaches, or even depression if it happens long enough. It could also show up as exhaustion, sleeplessness, or a sense that you are not in your body. If this happens over time, you can give your power away to the person who insists they know more about what is happening in you than you do.

Let's start off on your new journey with some writing prompts to help you assess if, how, and to whom you may be giving away your personal power. This is your way back to you.

- When you try to explain something about yourself, does someone tell you you're wrong?
- Who is this person?
- What does that feel like in your body?

- Do you distrust those physical signals?
- Do you believe people know better about your spiritual/emotional well-being than you do?
- What happens when the urge to express yourself to these people arises?
- What does that feel like in your body?
- Have you spoken up about an idea or perception that feels right to you but appears controversial to those around you?
- Do you shame yourself when someone tells you that you are wrong?

It's also important that you know when you might be denying another person's reality too. Here are some writing prompts that help you reflect on your own responses to others.

- Is there someone you struggle to hear when they express their pain?
- Do you take the position that yours is the only right way?
- How and to whom do you do that?
- How does that feel in your body?
- How can you slow down to listen to others' realities?

Over time, life reveals new ways of thinking, new views, new approaches. Stay curious about what comes to you. Stay open to possibilities. This does not put you in a position of weakness to listen to someone else whom you don't understand. Creating space to be curious brings you closer to your truth, which makes you powerful.

Journeying Within

The best—and possibly scariest—journey is within. It is the most rewarding one you will ever take because this journey is yours. You get to experience it. In fact, you are the only one who can. This is where the unique energy of your Soul resides. As you stay curious with the messages in your body, you start to access the deeper elements of yourself. Your Soul has been waiting this whole time to reconnect. This is joy. This is peace. This is empathy and compassion. Once you experience Soulful connection, you will find yourself equipped for any road ahead.

This may seem counter intuitive, but the way to your Soul is by attuning to the messages of your body. Your physical self is the cave entrance to the luminous echo that beckons you to enter. Your Soul will never steer you wrong, but first you must learn to listen for it. Don't let someone else manage your expedition by telling you what you need. Your Soul will tell you. Don't let doubt disconnect you from that inner guidance. That Soulful calling is the best GPS system you have.

There is an etheric playfulness to your Soul. It has integrated into your physical body and sometimes maneuvers it like a driver in a car. Sometimes, the wiring of the car overrides the driver. Staying curious to that interplay is how you can navigate your system.

Try the following exercise before you have any time to think about it.

EXERCISE
Capture the Moment

Stop what you are doing in this moment and notice how your body feels. Don't attempt to change or analyze anything. Just be curious. It doesn't matter if you are standing, sitting, or lying on your bed reading. Don't adjust anything.

- Notice the predominant energy in your body.
- Rest a palm there.
- Settle for a moment and connect to this area.
- Pull a breath toward where you are resting your hand.
- Be curious.
- Now, set your other hand on your heart.
- Pull a breath into your heart.
- Bring a few more breaths to the heart, then direct your attention back to where your first hand is resting.
- What are you noticing?
- Has the experience in your body shifted?
- Pay attention to the energy around both hands.
- What do you notice?
- Continue to stay here for as long as you like.
- Once you resume what you were doing, notice your body.
- What has changed?

Throughout that exercise, your system repatterned itself. You brought touch and kindness to your body. Through your vagus nerve and heart chakra, you brought safety to your body. Did you feel your mind ease?

This is the power you already have within you. Compassion and curiosity keep you present to yourself.

Mapping the Way

Even in utero, you were starting to feel strong connection to your body. Certainly, by the time you were born, your Soul was making connection to your physical self. The body is how you were able to decipher the human fullness of food, fear, and love as an infant. It was how you then learned to play with others and sense when you were not safe. Your body felt the pain of a scuffed knee as a toddler and hunger when you were ready to eat. It identified the distress of being left alone in a dark room at night, the anger of not being heard, and the love from a soft hug.

How many of your emotional experiences that expressed through your body got dismissed by others? Hard to tell. How many of these experiences now get dismissed by you? Learn to be curious about them again. Part of learning not to doubt the emotional signals your body wants to communicate is to not reason those signals away.[10]

Denying your own body signals may have started as missed cues from tired, well-intended parents or downright neglectful gestures from teachers, caretakers, or friends. How to disconnect from your physical self might have also been the mirrored behavior of the grown-ups around you. Remember that they received the same examples of how to detach as you did. They could not teach you something they did not know. One of the most challenging aspects of trauma is how the past can feel like it is present. This occurs because traumatic experiences are often not fully processed by the brain. Instead of being stored as past events, they remain active, with the body and mind responding as if the trauma is still

---

10. LeDoux, *The Emotional Brain*, 23.

occurring. This can result in flashbacks, intrusive thoughts, or intense emotional reactions triggered by reminders of the trauma.

For many, trauma feels like it exists outside the typical flow of time. The past is not experienced as something that has ended but rather as something ongoing and ever present. This can create a sense of being stuck, where the person feels trapped in their traumatic experience, unable to move forward because their body and mind are constantly reacting to the past as if it is the present. This phenomenon is often referred to as re-experiencing and is a key feature of conditions like post-traumatic stress disorder (PTSD).

Sheila's Story: Not Wanting to Look at the Blockages

When you are attuned to yourself, you can break cycles because you know what you need. When you're not present, you keep running in the same destructive patterns you used to survive as a child. Sometimes, those patterns seem so familiar they appear easy—except for when they're not. The story of my client Sheila is an example of that.

Sheila was a fifty-five-year-old mother of three teenagers. The day of our first session, I could hear Sheila coming down the hallway before I saw her. She didn't so much walk as she trotted. Her energy was high but chaotic. Her voice could be heard in the waiting room. She always dropped the things she was carrying, and her shoes would sometimes slip from her feet as she made her way toward me. Her curly brown hair would flop in her eyes, and she would blow the strands off her face. Sheila told me she was on an antidepressant and antianxiety medicine to get her through the day. She took various drugs to sleep since she reported this was the only way she could get to bed at a reasonable hour.

"I've told my doctor," she said during our first session, "none of these are working."

She was divorced but complained her "husband" would come to the house all the time. She was a teller at a local bank and grumbled that she kept getting passed up by the supervisor for administration roles. Sheila would get home from work exhausted but said she had to make dinner for her teenagers, do their laundry, and do her husband's laundry, too.

"It's like I'm not even divorced." she said. "He's over there five nights a week and sometimes sleeps in bed with me."

"And why is he there so often?" I asked.

"Oh." She pushed some hair off her face with her forearm. "He wants to see the kids."

I surmised the ex was there for all the great homemaking and sex Sheila was putting out, while he had his freedom to roam when he wanted to.

Her finances were also in shambles because she was financially pulling the weight for her children without the help of her former husband. When we discussed what setting limits might look like, she insisted she could not.

"My family would collapse if I didn't do things for them."

Me pointing out that fifteen-, sixteen-, and seventeen-year-olds were capable of at least cooking and cleaning seemed to go over her head. We discussed self-care; Sheila said she didn't have time. When I asked about her parents, she said her mother was still alive, and Sheila was the only one that drove her to appointments.

"Do the children drive?" I asked.

"Yes, but I don't trust them to drive Grammy around."

My client also complained she couldn't lose weight, that her hair was falling out, and she was exhausted in the mornings. She was a classic case of adrenal fatigue, but even when I approached her with this information, she didn't want to hear it. She spent the first several sessions charging herself up in a rage with complaints until she beamed with self-righteousness. Her cheeks flared red, and her breathing shortened.

While my initial assessment of Sheila didn't indicate any drug use and she didn't drink that much, I could only assume her raging at others got her through the day.

My intention with Sheila was to give her time to settle into a safe routine in our sessions and to honestly see if she was going to come back and be invested in any healing. I truly wanted her to feel heard. Raising her voice about things that were within her control that she stated were not told me she was desperately needing to be heard. However, the pattern of communication she was locked into was going to have to change if she was to experience peace.

During the third session, as Sheila was complaining about her boss again, I leaned forward and asked, "Where are you feeling that energy in your body right now?"

"What energy?" She looked stunned.

Her face was red, and I could see her heart thumping in her chest. I rested my hand on my heart and smiled at her. Sheila did the same, still looking a little confused.

After a long pause, she said, "Oh dear."

I nodded and continued to smile, not taking my gaze from her.

"This thing is gonna jump from my chest!" She patted her heart.

"Would you take in a slow breath?"

Sheila opened her mouth and loudly inhaled, then exhaled.

"Try this." I breathed in through my nose then slowly blew out of my mouth. "See how that feels."

She followed my slower breathing pace several times. I watched the color in her cheeks soften and her shoulders drop. Then I took my hand from my chest and smiled. "Whaddya think?"

"Wow." She shook her head. "I didn't know I could feel like that."

"So," I said. "You can feel even better than that over time. That was just a little glimpse into the future if we can do things a little differently."

Sheila looked over at me and got teary-eyed. "Please don't leave me," she said. Her voice sounded small and young. This was the first time I had heard the slightest bit of vulnerability.

"I won't leave you," I said.

She cleared her throat and nodded. Her face paled. "Yes," she said. "I just don't want anyone else to leave."

"Let's do this together," I said. "I don't want you to feel as bad as you are feeling. We will go slow, okay?"

"Okay," she said. "I'm just used to being in charge. It scares me not to be."

"I hear that," I said. "I'm not trying to take charge of you. I'm trying to give you some ways to help you have some actual charge over yourself."

She blinked. "Oh, wow. I don't think anyone has ever put it that way before."

For the first time in a session, Sheila talked about her father and his erratic, violent episodes that seemed to come out of nowhere when she was a child. She said she would hide under the bed when all her other tactics to please him failed.

"That's where I would stuff cookies and candy," she said. "It was my only refuge some days."

Her mother worked long hours and sometimes two jobs. Sheila felt unprotected by the only person in the house that didn't rage at her. She wondered if her mother was working so much just to avoid her husband.

"He was just a moody bastard," she said. "You never knew when it was coming. He didn't drink. At least if he did, I didn't notice. Then my brother started acting like him. It was like walking into a fireworks warehouse with a lit match." She lowered her head. "Then I married a man like them, ironically, just to escape them." As Sheila spoke, her face grew expressionless, and she started to slump.

I pointed to my window. Outside was a walking path and a lake. "Sounds random, but do you want to go for a walk?" I asked.

She looked up, surprised I was even in the room, then said, "Okay."

What Sheila didn't know, which she would come to learn through our trauma work, was that she had dissociated from her body as she was talking. The slow walk around the lake would engage her in some activity that would bring her back safely into her body.

My initial work with her, I explained, was to get her to understand and identify the deactivated response she was having. Dissociating when she either talked about or experienced a lack of safety wasn't a character flaw. It was her nervous system trying to keep her safe like it did when her father raged. We started working with some ways for her to move differently. I helped her understand what the body does in response to stress, and we mapped out what her exclusive patterns were with assessments. Before we even worked through the traumatic memories, I had to help Sheila be present and feel safe enough in her body to do that. This is work that I see as very collaborative and supportive, which establishes safety in the working relationship.

Sheila's ability to find balance in her body took a while. Her rushed, chaotic pace, as if she was running from something, kept her off balance. She would have a burst of what is called a flight response as she got to my office followed by a moment of shutting down or freezing. As getting her to reconnect with her body was going to be a slow go, I started with basics.

"Look at the ducks in the water." I pointed to the lake when we would walk.

"Oh, nice," she said. Her tone was distracted, like she wanted to get this over with. I noticed her fumbling with her phone in her pocket.

"What do you feel in your body right now?"

She looked away as if wanting an escape. "Nervousness."

"You're safe," I said.

This statement settled her a bit. She stared at the ducklings that were swimming behind their mother. "Oh," she said. "They're really cute."

"Notice where you feel that cuteness in your body." I put my hand on my heart to model what that might look like.

Sheila looked for a while longer, then rested her hand on her belly. "Kinda warm here."

"Nice," I said. I waited a minute, then started to walk again. "Wanna take our shoes off?"

"You're kidding, right?" This surprised her. "I dunno. I've never done that before."

It was summer, so I was wearing sandals. I slipped them off and stood in the grass.

"I'm kind of embarrassed about my feet," she said.

"Oh no," I said. "I don't want you to feel bad."

However, she took off her heavy leather shoes. Her nails had not been clipped in a while, and her feet were peeling. Sheila looked up with an embarrassed grin. "I just don't take care of them."

"Have you ever had a pedicure?"

She shook her head. "Never have the time."

I laughed. "Let's put that on your treatment plan. Not for cosmetic reasons but because it feels awesome when you do it. You deserve to be touched in caring ways."

She teared up and didn't say anything for a while. Both of us moved our toes and dug our heels into the cool grass. The walk back was slower and calmer. I was quiet and gave Sheila the space to reflect as she seemed to be working something through.

"I have moved so fast all my life," she said at the end of the session, "just to please others, that I have never slowed down enough to feel grass beneath my feet."

The next week Sheila came into the office and slipped off her new shoes. She wiggled her toes and happily displayed her red nail polish.

"Nice!" I laughed.

"I can't believe it, but I feel a little different." She shook her head. "No one has ever touched my feet before. There was something weirdly"—she paused—"grounding in that. I even walk a little slower because I don't want to mess up my toes."

We laughed and decided pedicures would be a monthly treatment plan "to-do." Sheila and I worked weekly for over a year. Eventually, she said she wanted to process some of the scary events from her childhood since she felt she could be present enough for them.

I used various eye movement techniques designed to reprocess traumatic memories from the brain and nervous system with her. Her startle responses disappeared. She slept through the night. She said she felt calm enough to take a full breath in stressful places like work.

Sheila also said she was able to develop some insight and compassion for her brother, who was suffering with the same mental health issues her father had. "However"—she raised a finger—"compassion with boundaries; isn't that what you say? He won't be invited for Thanksgiving dinner anytime soon."

The evolution of how Sheila learned to be present in her life was moving. Sheila eventually started meditation and yoga classes with no prompting from me, as I feel that is something a client must be curious to do for themselves. She was still a doer, so the class gave her some structure and guidance. Yoga movement also allowed her more regular practice to access her emotions since she felt comfortable in her body now. This also started to help Sheila set limits with her children, her mother, and her ex. Because she was now comfortable in her felt experience, she could sense her inner truth, and she listened. Sheila learned to identify her own needs and care for herself without guilt. She found safety enough to access her peace.

Sheila finally found herself, and it wasn't through meeting the needs of others. The following are two exercises I did with Sheila.

EXERCISE
Earth to Sky Zip

Anytime you are not feeling in your body or you need a quick movement to ground and energize yourself, try this Earth to Sky Zip. This brings your whole body into play. It reaches down to connect to the ground and extends high to connect upward. This movement "zips" up the energy of your chakras, engages the mobility in your vagus, and connects that electromagnetic energy of the ground to the heavens. When you are feeling stressed, it balances. If you are tired, it will invigorate. It feels like an energetic boundary around those parts of your body that can be drained. Zipping pulls things in and keeps them in place.

Before you do this, check in with your body. How do you feel? This is a nice way to gauge the before and after of the exercise.

- Stand with feet shoulder width apart.
- Rest hands by sides.
- Slightly bend knees in an effort to have feet firmly connected to the ground.
- Bend down and touch fingers (or palms if you can) to the ground.
- Stay there for a few seconds.
- Slowly, scoop the earth's energy into your hands and start to stand.
- As if you are pulling a large zipper up, move your hands from the ground upward.
- Keep zipping over your groin, up the belly, and over the heart, throat, and middle of the face.
- Reach both hands upward as you zip up over your head.
- Then reach as high as you can into the air and stretch your whole body toward the sky.
- Do this at least three times.

How are you experiencing your energy now? Do this exercise anytime you need to actively center yourself.

EXERCISE
Writing Prompt: Retracing Your Steps

Do you know the difference between a thought and an emotion? They are both so rapid-fire in your system that they intertwine and feel like one big ball. If you slow down and retrace your thinking steps, you can reveal the emotions that stir behind your thoughts. Differentiating a thought from a feeling may be a foreign (and scary) concept. Many of us were never shown that there is a difference. However, knowing when you are thinking and how this is affecting your emotions can change everything. First, this helps you understand what is occurring in your inner world. This way you can own your reality. Then, knowing how your thoughts affect your emotions helps you communicate better. Your thinking steps have to slow down so you can observe.

Let's try this writing prompt to see where you have traveled with a thought. This will help you. Start by filling in the blanks to this sentence.

Find a recent situation involving a conflict with a person that may still feel charged in your body.

In the first blank, write the person's name.

In the second blank, write out what you think of them or their intention regarding the interaction.

In the third, write what they did or said and what you think their intention was.

I think _____ is _____ because they

_____.

As you look at that sentence, I bet the memory of what happened feels strong in your body. Check in and notice where you feel the energy. Without attempting to put a narrative to it, just put your hand on the energy right now.

- Breathe into that energy.
- Sit with it.
- Continue to breathe.
- Let that energy know you are honoring it.
- Let it know you understand it is there.
- Keep breathing into it.

Look at the following words. I want you to circle the ones that most closely define your energy right now. You can come up with more. These are just prompts to get you started.

Sad   Lonely   Terrified   Mad   Annoyed   Glad

Are you surprised by what you circled?

If you circled *Mad*, continue to sit with that energy. Ask the energy if it has anything else it wants to share. Just be with it a while. Is there another emotion there? Perhaps more vulnerability? Sadness? Loneliness? Fear?

Now, rewrite this sentence.

When _____ did _____ what I thought was _____. What I feel is _____, and it is located in my _____.

Thinking is based on a framework of past experiences. It pulls from old datasets and more than likely has a well-trod pathway in your brain. Those thoughts and beliefs are sent from your brain down to your nervous system and stir emotions.

Your brain doesn't want you to feel vulnerable, so many times its first impulse is to generate anger. That is why I suggest you sit with the anger for a while to notice if there is anything behind it. Once Sheila was able to do this, she understood her life was full of complexity that she didn't have to fear.

Learning to Drive

Like your car, your human system is made of various components. All parts need to function well together to get you where you want to go. Start considering you are a whole. You are not broken up into multiple systems that work independently from each other. One structure supports the next. This way, you will pay attention differently.

Your body is constantly reading, constantly relating to external and internal stimuli, and sending this information to other parts of your "engine." Pay attention to what your body is communicating and honor the experiences, just as you would listen to the information on your GPS or lights on your dashboard. It displays things you need to know. When you can see yourself in this way, you can apply curiosity. Attuning lets you slow, still, or move. It helps you turn your wheel and head in another direction if necessary. When you honor the subtle (or not so subtle) energies in your body and become adept at gauging them, you develop advance driving skills.

Sometimes you have to retrace your route and go back to that fork in the road to take the other path—the healing path. There is no failure in that. Think of a metaphorical pit stop on a racetrack. There is only strength when you can drive your car back to where it started and tune up with tools that support you. So, let's break down some of the features that make up your human experience.

Body

When you experience a thought, you feel it in your body. When your nervous system responds, you feel it in your body. When you feel emotion, you feel it in your body. Sometimes, these layers of experience are all sensed at once. This is called affect.[11] Affect is not a bad thing. It is truly the way you are designed to pay attention. Your body leads you with several sonar-like systems that help guide the way and reveal themselves through your affective experience.

If you have been conditioned to doubt your physical messaging centers (we all have), then tuning in to your body for information is a hard concept to grasp. If you have been physically or emotionally hurt—especially in childhood—connecting to your body seems downright frightening. Your internal wiring through your nervous system may have even developed responses to keep you from connecting.

Within your body, you have a brain. Though it might feel like it at times, it's not really the enemy; its thinking just gets misguided based on previous data. Know that the brain is just one part of your internal messaging center. Like the dashboard indicators in a car, the brain is a vital measure of how the other systems are functioning. When that system goes out, it is hard to know how the rest of the vehicle is doing. When those lights are working the way they should, you can trust the data to help you move forward. The brain's wiring, or nerve fibers, contribute to this communication.

There are twelve nerve fibers in your brain that signal your senses; they are called cranial nerves. They are listed with roman numerals in anatomy books.[12] Your vagus nerve is the tenth of those cranial nerves (CNX). It runs from the brain down both sides of the body and attaches to all the major organs that help you— among other things—breathe, digest, and manage your heart rate.

---

11. Dana, *Anchored*, 20.
12. Felten and O'Banion and Summo Maida, *Netter's Atlas of Neuroscience*, 270.

Your nervous system and brain are the wiring you don't see but you most certainly feel. The vagus nerve signals up to your brain and receives messages back from your brain, as both are constantly evaluating if you are safe.[13] Because the vagus nerve is part of your "security system," it constantly scans for potential threats to your well-being.[14] It stores memories of times you were or were not safe, and these experiences are also patterned into the organs it communicates with.

If the brain and vagus nerve interpret a threat, it fires off signals to the major organs of your body. Such an experience is considered a visceral one. Have you ever felt a stomachache when the boss got angry? Do you struggle with a rapid heart rate when you are in rush hour traffic? Does your swallowing stop or increase when you get scared? Do you struggle to listen well to others when you are stressed?

When you feel danger, your body can go into overdrive or even shut down. Both can feel overpowering. The intensity of that messaging is generally why so many people distrust connecting to their body for guidance, as they haven't learned to differentiate emotions from a physiological response.

When your mind and nervous system perceive safety, you barely notice this gauge because your body experiences a stasis or balance. You are calm and connected. Your heart rate and blood pressure lower; your breathing is more rhythmic. You feel comforted by the people and places around you.

---

13. Porges and Porges, *Our Polyvagal World*, 47.
14. Porges, *Polyvagal Safety*, 81.

Mind

Let's get back to the thinking part for a moment. Mind, in this case, is not the brain. Mind is the meaning you form and the reality you make about your life utilizing the functions of your brain.[15] However, that brain of yours has a tendency toward a negativity bias.[16] This means it leans into remembering the bad things over the good in an effort to keep you safe. This is a built-in protective measure that kept your ancestors alive. They learned where the dangers were so they didn't travel those routes. They remembered poisonous plants and scanned with eyes, ears, and intuitive senses for animals lurking in the high grasses with that negativity bias.

This trending toward looking for harm is built into your DNA. It forms the reality of your life if you are not aware of it. Negative thinking patterns become so common they feel like truth. Thoughts fire off signals in your body. They might even bring a momentary burst of energy as hormones kick in. Perceptions of fear, cynicism, or judgment are sent down to your nervous system just as rapidly as stored memories based on these perceptions are sent up—reinforcing that negative bias. Mind is the lens by which you see people, places, and things.

How and what you believed in your younger years can get entangled into a present-day reality. That may perpetuate old pain. How and what you believe now, however, can be reshaped as new experiences unfold for you. Staying in present-time awareness through mindfulness practices is one of the healing tools you can use to reshape your life. Every one of your present moments of safety builds on the next. This makes room for the more flexible practice of curiosity and kindness.

---

15. Siegel, *Mindsight*, 12.
16. Fisher, *Healing the Fragmented Selves of Trauma Survivors*, 37.

Community

Community is the way you participate with the people and places in your life. Your world can be made up of intimate relationships, coworkers who share space but not personal connection, acquaintances, and the town you live in or the town you grew up in as well as the greater world. Perceptions of how safe these people are to you register in your system in ways you might not notice. Sometimes your communities are not safe due to family dynamics, racial inequities or socioeconomic disparities, or violence. These are true moments of lack of safety. How you feel in your body as you engage within your communities is an indicator of how safe you feel within yourself.

If you are with safe community but cannot feel that in your body, that is a result of your nervous system struggling with past harms and not a personality flaw. Notice if experiences of threat in your body are coming from present-day experiences or past trauma. Some breathing techniques in this chapter may help you to manage this.

The Chakras and Energy Fields

Sensations of safety with others extend beyond your internal experience and transmit outside of your body. This explains why you can sometimes feel a person before you see them or why as you are thinking of them they call you. That etheric energy field that transmits communication is impossible to measure. Is it in you or outside of you? Is it an extension of Soul energy that makes up an Indra's net of connection?[17] Is it an electromagnetic sphere that includes the earthly biosphere? Perhaps all of these or none

---

17. Robertson, *Indra's Net*, 76.

of these. Regardless, you experience these psychic transmissions whether you consciously tune in or not.

Think of that chill you get when a loved one passes and you didn't know it at the time, that calm experience that your grandmother is standing behind you and sending love. Because these experiences are so personal, this information is exiled by institutions (including many religious ones) to the woo-woo corner of human interaction where it sits in shame. Even in my highly intuitive field, we clinicians carefully dance around the woo-woo parts for fear of not being solid in our skill sets. Thankfully change is upon us. It's not a balanced human experience to have to choose between a tangible or a subjective camp. Humans are both. We don't have to be only intuition or measurement. Your healing is measured by the subjective changes you experience.

Your chakras, which are concentrated points of energy along your body, extend and connect with others' experiences. They are both generative and receptive, taking in information while sending out.[18] I see them align with the vagus nerve as I work with clients. Your vagus nerve is also generative and receptive. I encourage clients to listen to their energy centers, as those spots provide opportunities to access old memories or receive profound new insights. The more you can slow down and take note of your energetic experiences, the more psychological information for healing you can connect to.

People carry old patterning in their body and that naturally seeps out into the etheric field. Some energies are not well intended. Some energies carry unintended pain. How well a person has healed from their past by alleviating traumatic patterning from their

---

18. Motoyama, *Theories of the Chakras*, 268.

nervous system shifts not only internally but extends outward and affects humanity.

Soul

Studying how the Soul gets into and chooses the body is the work of past-life regressionists and those who have had near-death experiences.[19] Past-life regressionists or life-between-life regressionists use hypnotherapy as a way to guide clients back to the early memories of this life or other lives they have experienced. According to the life-between-life work that has been done by Michael Newton and the Michael Newton Institute,[20] the Soul generally chooses and takes on a body several months after conception and still in utero (depending on the Soul's desired lesson). They also have learned of Souls that wait until after the body has been born.

The regressionists are finding the way the Soul enters the body is by way of the chakras and frequently the crown chakra. As the Soul integrates with the body, it starts to activate through the brain and vagus nerve. This information has been compiled through decades of Michael Newton's and researchers of the Michael Newton Institute's work. Researchers write that Souls choose an amnesiac barrier in life. They report that it is within that mystery we learn our deepest lessons. In other words, if we knew why we were here, we wouldn't learn anything.

When you hear that researchers are finding your Soul light drives your embodied self, does this change anything for you? If so, how does this change things? Does this help you tend to yourself with deeper awareness? More kindness? Certainly more curiosity.

---

19. Weiss, *Only Love Is Real*, 25; Alexander, *Proof of Heaven*.
20. Newton, *Journey of Souls*.

Perhaps you can more skillfully manage the human navigation signals in your body.

Know, too, that Soul does not reflect a belief system; it echoes its own inimitable energy. Your inner truth can get lost in the noise of humanity, but you can certainly find your way back to it. Healing your human parts clears the way.

Remember When?

Do you remember when you were young and moved your body in intuitive ways? You would swing your arms and kick your feet and roll on the ground just because it felt good. Remember the breaths you would take? They were full and loud, and they rounded out your belly. Did you breathe and even rest your hands on your belly, enjoying the warm expansiveness of your tummy? Until you were told differently, you took a full breath that filled your whole torso. Even at birth, your stomach filled with air. This is an intuitive form of breathing that we forgot over the years. As stressors piled, we started pulling shorter breaths into the lungs until our lungs barely filled with air.

While throwing yourself on the ground and rolling around in joy might get you fired at the office (save that one for when you're at home), you can certainly return to the experience of a childlike breath in public with no one questioning you.

When you do this, you are more grounded and joyful. That's because when air fills your body, your internal organs and nervous system get more of what they need. This is called diaphragmatic breathing. It's a breath massage of sorts.

By the way, unless otherwise noted, all the breathing exercises in this book will be done breathing in through your nose and slowly out your mouth. This is for several reasons. The first is that nose breathing screens toxins, as the hairs in your nose act as a filtration system. The second is that nose breathing pulls oxygen into the tissues of your system more efficiently.[21] The process releases nitric oxide, which increases carbon dioxide, which is needed for oxygen.

To get you started on this path to reclaiming your ability to be present to your body, let's start with breathing like you're a child again. I have several approaches for you. Here are the first two.

EXERCISE
Breathe Like a Baby Again

For the first breathing exercise, play around with how it feels to soften and expand your belly. If you can't do this at first, it's okay. We all got so conditioned to tightening and slumping that we lost the capacity for our body to properly do its job. Full-belly breathing, or diaphragmatic breathing, engages the whole diaphragm.

Using half the capacity of our lungs doesn't even make sense. Imagine working out but only using half of your leg or arm muscles. So, let's reclaim a full childlike breath by regularly practicing diaphragmatic breathing. Once this comes back to you, it will be natural because you were already doing this once upon a time.

This full-belly breathing takes the pressure off so many parts of your body. The upper regions of your shoulders and neck work overtime just to pull a breath into the top of your lungs. Your neck carries a lot of pressure when you only take short breaths. Maybe you even experience headaches.

---

21. "Diaphragmatic Breathing."

Breathing deeply, into the full expanse of your lungs, creates a whole new world for you.

Straighten your spine and lift your chin a little by looking straight ahead. Sitting straight is not being rigid. It's making room for the body parts you cannot see. That room is for the vagal nerve fibers that innervate your breathing. It opens space for the upper regions of your nasal cavity and mouth. It allows for the larynx and pharynx—which are part of your respiratory and digestive tract—to get involved. Because you are breathing deeply, you are activating the lower portions of your respiratory tract. The bronchi and bronchial tubes carry oxygen deep within the lungs and help with gas exchange. That oxygen releases into the bloodstream.

First Baby Breath

A full breath changes everything, so make way for a new physiological experience that will create a new affective one.

- Sit comfortably in your chair.
- Relax your shoulders and chest.
- Soften your stomach muscles.
- Draw the breath into your nose.
- Pull your breath down into your stomach below your belly button.
- Imagine the stomach muscles pulling the air down.
- Softly exhale through your mouth.
- Notice the sensations.
- What are you thinking?
- Do you feel those thoughts in your body?
- Keep going.
- Notice how you are speaking to yourself as you breathe.

- Be gentle on yourself if you struggle with softening your stomach.
- Notice the air as it fills your belly.
- Be aware of all sensations as breathing into your tummy becomes natural again.
- Notice the sensations in your belly.
- Continue to notice the muscles around your arms, shoulders, and neck.
- How do you feel in your body?
- Do any memories from childhood arise?
- Is this the first time you have had so much air fill your body?
- What thoughts are here?
- What emotions are here?
- How do you feel in your seat right now?

Second Baby Breath

We are going to see if these belly breaths can be so expansive that they soften your ribs and make space in the intercostal muscles between the ribs. What a great way to make room for your digestive organs.

Continue to sit in your chair for support as you practice this.

- Relax in your chair.
- Soften your belly muscles.
- Notice your shoulders and arms.
- Be curious about your neck muscles, your jaw, and your head.
- Draw a breath in through your nose.
- Imagine the flexible rib cage of bone, fascia, and intercoastal muscles expanding.

- Softly exhale through your mouth.
- Breathe deeper into your belly like you did before.
- Let the breath move sideways into your rib cage.
- Keep going.
- Notice.
- How does this change the earlier belly breath?
- Are you using your lungs differently?
- What are you observing about your torso movement?
- How does this feel in your body?
- Keep gently drawing the breath into your rib cage.
- Any old memories?
- What are your thoughts?
- Do you feel them in your body?
- See yourself as making room for the intestines, lungs, and heart.
- Keep going.
- Notice how your body feels as it experiences more air and expansion.
- Draw the breath in slowly and exhale just as slowly.
- What thoughts are here?
- What emotions are here?
- How does your body feel in the chair?

When you are driving, sitting at your desk, walking, standing, doing dishes, or any other routine tasks, do your diaphragmatic breathing. Initially, this might be more air than you're used to, so take it slow and listen to your body.

Affect

Did you notice throughout those exercises that I asked you how you felt in your body when breathing? Did you also notice that I asked you what emotions were present? I even asked what you thought and how you felt in your body as you thought. How you think can create a rapid meaning or memory that stirs your nervous system into a response. These physical sensations, which stem from various sources, can all be considered "affect," or that felt experience in your body.

Neuroscientists study the brain to determine affective expression.[22] Sociologists and philosophers study affect from the perspective of how it affects the wider culture.[23] Trauma therapists make room for affect in sessions. We help the clients develop awareness and presence around it. We treat affect as the window into healing, though as we all know, breathing into affect and staying curious about it takes time and trust because more than likely affect has overwhelmed you in the past.

You can also say that affect drives more of your choices than you may realize. Since affect can range from pleasant to uncomfortable to downright insufferable within seconds, we respond quickly to it. We all have old techniques to avoid what we perceive as emotional pain. If the affect is pleasant, we allow it. When that affect is more difficult, we look for diversions. Those diversions can be numbing through drugs and alcohol, engaging in risky sex, binging, buying, keeping too busy—the list goes on. These thoughts and the behaviors stemming from them are rapid and habitual.

---

22. Damasio, *Descartes' Error*.
23. Berlant, *Cruel Optimism*.

How do you understand your affective experience? First, increase awareness about what and where you are feeling your affect. Then notice that moment when you want to lean forward and do something. Don't shame yourself. Just notice. Be curious.

Part of healing is to reconnect you to that childlike ease you had at one time. Knowing your current affective state at any given moment is important to reclaiming a sense of safety in your body—even if in that moment your affect doesn't feel safe. You felt difficult affect as a child. We all did. However, many times back then you moved in intuitive ways that naturally helped that energy along. Those "hits and tension" are your body's neurobiological mechanisms that have been activated.[24] The most hopeful part of understanding this is that you have the power to shift it.

Arousal States and Breath

Have you ever been waiting to do a presentation and found yourself breathing quick, short breaths? Did you hold your breath after a deep exhale? Did you slowly release that breath? Of those, which felt the best?

When you can manage your affective state through breath, you increase your overall ability to calm your nervous system and develop what is referred to as vagal tone.[25] Vagal tone is how easily you can restore your heart back to a calmer state.

Your breaths send caring messages to your nervous system (or not). Deeper, calmer breaths reestablish that childlike ease you once had in your body. Studies have shown that singers and vocal performers have very strong heart rate variability—slower beats between beats—because of the control they have over their vocal

---

24. Allen, *Coping with Trauma*, 58–59.
25. Porges, *Polyvagal Perspectives*, 52.

quality.[26] Other studies indicated choir singers' heart rates synchronize as they sing. This body of yours has so much ability to heal itself with breath.

There are two arousal states that feel uncomfortable. One is overstimulation. It is a dysregulated experience coming from your sympathetic branch of the vagus and puts you on high alert. This is where your nervous system gets hyper-aroused. This might look like agitation, anger, or being short-tempered. Hyper-arousal puts you in a state of fighting or wanting to escape. Sometimes both. Whole communities can stay in hyper-arousal, and many media outlets even stimulate this in their audience to get a response. Are you aware of when you feel hyper-aroused?

The other end of that arousal spectrum is the experience of shutting down. This is when the nervous system is hypo-aroused, which means you are not fully connected to your body. You may be looking down from above or experiencing a haze. You could not be hearing the people in the room even though your body looks like it is listening. In trauma terms, this is called dissociation. On some levels we all do it. Are you aware of when you feel hypo-aroused?

The first thing to do is to bring awareness to your arousal state. Are you feeling disconnected or so stimulated that you can't stay seated? Be inquisitive. Know that these states ebb and flow. This is part of the lived human experience through the nervous system. Be present to the moment. This is where you are safe because this is what you can control.[27] Determining your arousal state will help you determine which of the following breathing approaches your body needs.

---

26. Vickhoff et al., "Music Structure Determines Heart Rate Variability of Singers."
27. Goldstein, *Mindfulness*, 101.

EXERCISE
Breathing In for Energy

The in breath increases oxygen in your bloodstream, especially when you can pull that breath deep into your lungs. The in breath stimulates the body and raises the heart rate. It actives the mobility branch of your vagus. When you are in need of reconnecting and invigorating your body, use deeper in breaths. Hold, then a use a slightly more rapid out breath.

As always, these breathing exercises have variations depending on your needs. Pay attention to how you feel as you do this exercise.

- Take in a breath through your nose and fill the lungs as far as you can.
- Hold for a time that feels right for you.
- Release the breath with a slightly faster pace than the intake.
- Do this as many times as you need.
- How do you feel?
- What are you noticing in your body?

EXERCISE
Breathing Out for Calm

The out breath increases heart rate variability. Increasing the time between beats means your overall heart rate slows and calms the rest of your body. Longer heart rate variability is optimal. This slow exhale engages the fibers of the vagus that manage this. It expels carbon dioxide in that necessary exchange of gases that fuel the bloodstream.

- Sit in a relaxing position.
- Take in a breath to fill the lungs just enough to reach full capacity.
- Hold if it feels right.
- Imagine you are about to breathe into a flute through your mouth.
- Release the breath slowly.
- Keep the exhale going as if you are breathing into that flute for as long as you can.
- Imagine you are expelling all breath from your lungs before taking in another breath.
- Continue this until you feel a shift.
- How do you feel?
- What are you noticing?

So, Then, What *Is* an Emotion?

How do you discern an emotion from a neurobiological response in your body? Did you know there was a difference? Does the idea of feeling emotions frighten you? Don't let it. It is good and right to open to emotions.

Emotions get a bad rap. Emotion is felt in the body, but it's an experience of energy and movement. Carl Jung wrote that emotions are expressions of the unconscious mind and Soul.[28] There may never be words to fully describe the expanse of energy the Soul possesses; however, when Soul is at the forefront of an emotional experience, there is an undeniable depth.

When you can make room, emotions guide you. They may be an inexplicable longing for an experience your mind doesn't

---

28. Jung, *Man and his Symbols.*

understand or an undisturbed knowing about what is right. Emotion is not a brittle experience that makes you want to shut down or run. An emotional experience is a vast one. Emotions are form and color, a full spectrum of Soul energy that even includes anger—sometimes profoundly so.

The energy of Soul is immeasurable because, of course, Soul is an envoy from the universe.[29] Even with loss, Soulful emotions have depth. The edges are not sharp but fill the body with profundity. The emotional experience of grief is powerful and palpable. Enigmatic. It may run deep or sit in stillness.

Soulful expression does not create the same forceful impact on your body that a survival response does. Survival responses come from your neurobiology. They are intense and "punchy," which is how I describe them to my clients. They rev you up or shut you down. Soulful emotion fills you with energy that expands and contracts, softening and filling. As Jung says, the soul is "the life principle, the essence of everything alive."[30]

Emotion Desires Expression, Trauma Seeks Healing

Sometimes it's hard to sort through a deep emotional response when something awful and out of the ordinary happens. An unexpected death is one of those intense experiences that confuses your system. What is the effect of trauma on your body versus what is an emotional longing? Sometimes, the traumatic grief must be processed before that deeper missing can even be visited.

The trauma around loss is usually about the last moments of a person (or a pet's) death. How they died or the images refueling in your brain about that death can permanently haunt your system.

---

29. Hunt, *Infinite Mind*, 296.
30. Jung, *Archetypes and the Collective Unconscious.*

Sorting through the trauma of loss takes time and is helped along with a good trauma therapist. They will understand that it is not the grief that needs to be alleviated but the stuck data points in your system that keep you in the last moments of that death. When you can help your nervous system deprogram, you can eventually develop a new kind of bond with your loved one.

Summary

You are constructed of intricately woven parts that make up a whole. You are a simple being that possesses great complexity. The internal life force of your Soul is more profound than your human mind can comprehend. Your physical body is key to heeding your Soul. Become aware of how your vagus nerve communicates for you and tend to the messages it whispers through the etheric energy of your chakras. The energy of your Soul drives the human messaging systems of your vagus nerve and brain like a driver steers a car. That internal light is the light that extends outside of you through your chakras. This is the lived tension you balance. Listening in this way takes practice and work. You ebb and flow. You are at times far more physical and sometimes far more in touch with your wisdom light. Certainly, as you restore equanimity in your nervous system, that Soul shines through more easily. As a result, the path gets a tad easier to travel.

Differentiating a thought from a feeling is a foreign concept if you were never shown how. Given your brain has a natural negativity bias that is constantly searching for danger, untethered thinking stirs your nervous system into protective mode. These physical sensations, which are innervated from the three branches of your vagus nerve, are considered affect. *Affect* is a general term meaning felt experiences. Approaching affective states with curiosity and not skepticism is the way. When you can manage your affective states through breath, you increase your ability to calm your nervous system, specifically your vagus nerve. Managed breathing sends messages of safety to your nervous system and helps reestablish that childlike ease you once had.

There is a difference between emotions and the affect experienced in your body when you don't feel safe. Emotions are expressed from the higher, wiser energy of your Soul. They are softer, even when those emotions are sadness or loneliness. Be gentle with yourself as you open to the different experiences. Don't hand over your personal power to someone else so they can decide and choose your experiences for you. This is your life. Stand in your power by knowing your personal truth. There is great learning to this living and even greater learning from healing.

CHAPTER 2

ALL WHO WANDER ARE NOT LOST

⎯⎯●⎯⎯⎯⎯⎯●⎯⎯

The vagus nerve and chakras simultaneously galvanize, though it would seem the vagus leads the charge more than the chakras shift the state of the vagus.

When the body experiences distress and shuts down, chakra energy seems to tighten or close. If that immobility releases the bowels, the lower chakras overactivate. When the nervous system signals danger and mobilizes, energy courses through the chakras closest to the adrenals. In a state of calm, chakra energy seems to flow in all areas of the body.

The chakras and vagus nerve work in tandem. Over two thousand years of Eastern wisdom bears this out. The ancient yogis described the chakric energy that flows along the body as aligning with nerve centers.[31] Yogis have also associated organs and their functions with the quality of the chakras. As you are learning, your vagus, the largest autonomic nerve branch, connects and communicates with the major organs of your body. We are just starting to be able to measure what the ancients knew.

There is one more vital part to this schematic, so I have to back up some. It's really the start of it all. Nothing—no nervous system or mental processing—can intelligently charge if your Soul is not dancing around in there somewhere. It is your Soul that lights up

---

31. Avalon, *The Serpent Power*, 103.

all your bodily hardware. It is your Soul that directs its luminosity through the fibers of your being. It is your Soul's vitality that beams like a sentinel—sending messages and awaiting replies—through what we call your chakras. When you feel the energy along the core of your body, you are experiencing the energy of your Soul.

Take a look at this diagram and see if it helps you understand the schematic. The Soul enters the body, and it integrates with the human "hardware" of the brain and nervous system, which reflects outward along and from the body.

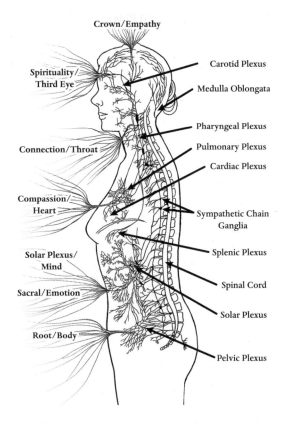

Figure 2: Chakras, the Vagus Nerve, and the Soul – Schema

You don't have to subscribe to my term *Soul*. Call it "mind energy" or "inner light." Call it the essence that is here that eventually leaves the body. In *The Egyptian Book of the Dead*, the ancient Egyptians referred to Soul as "ka" and the personality as "ba," separating the psychological aspects that form identity from the inner essence. The Internal Family Systems model discovered that while we develop many personality aspects to help us manage and protect ourselves through life's stressors, we have a higher, wiser Self that, when accessed, reparents these burdened ego parts of us.[32]

Regardless of how you term it, there is one thing no one on the planet can argue: When that energy that seems uniquely us leaves the body, there is no more intelligent functioning in the system. No chakras, no auras, no energy fields hang around once the Soul leaves. No nervous system responds in any intelligent way. This is the part we humans seem to dance around. When that vehicle we came here in stops running, the lights go out.

So, let's keep learning about that vehicle your Soul chose to drive. Like all cars, we need to perform upkeep. If we don't, that car starts running us. No matter how hard we pump the brakes, if we haven't maintained them, the car could crash. Cars and their electrical systems override the drivers' intentions all the time. The systems in that body of yours need regular attention. You have to know when these parts are not working well in order to know what to fix. How else will you keep trucking along on your journey?

What Is Your Vagus Nerve?

Vagus is Latin for "wandering." For centuries the medical community surmised these lengthy strands of nerve fiber were doing

---

32. Schwartz, *No Bad Parts*.

just that. However, the more we advance in our scientific and spiritual learning, the more it becomes evident that no part of the human design is random. The vagus is the longest branch in your autonomic nervous system (ANS), which is part of your central nervous system (CNS). For clarity, the autonomic nervous system *automatically* keeps your respiratory, cardiac, and digestive structures going. It also, according to polyvagal theory, tracks for safety.[33]

The vagus nerve branches out from the base of your brain along the jugular foramen (an opening at the base of the skull) and runs along the neck, the carotid artery, and jugular vein. It travels down to the upper respiratory and digestive branches of the larynx, pharynx, and esophagus into the thorax cavity to connect with the chest, heart, and lungs. Its bilateral branches extend into the large and small intestines, liver, gallbladder, and pancreas. This nerve may appear to wander, but it is by no means lost. It knows exactly what it's doing and where it's going. This great communicator connects your brain to your liver through hepatic vagal branches.[34] It affects hormones and blood pressure, manages inflammatory factors, and helps convert glycogen to glucose. The health of your gut—which assists with brain functioning—is a primary contributor to how well the vagus does its job.[35]

---

33. Porges, *Polyvagal Theory*, 11.
34. Felten, O'Banion, and Summo Maida, *Netter's Atlas of Neuroscience*, 223.
35. Rosenberg, *Accessing the Healing Power of the Vagus Nerve*, 27.

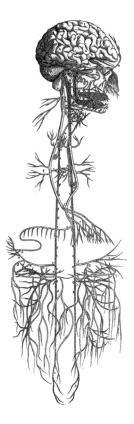

Figure 3: Vagus Nerve

★ ★ ★

There are two components of the vagus nerve that align with the messages from your chakras' energy flow. The subdiaphragmatic branch is below the respiratory diaphragm. This branch connects to the esophagus, gastric branches and extends to the intestines. These branches are not myelinated, which means there is no fatty coating around them. This is helpful to know because the information traveling along your digestive tract is slower and can be felt beyond the organ(s). An example is when a stomachache becomes a backache for no apparent reason. Many times, because of this generalized discomfort, we want to reject this area of our body. When we do chakra work, we get particularly suspicious of the energy centers that align here.

The supradiaphragmatic branch, which is above the solar plexus region, encompasses the organs from the lungs and heart upward. It is myelinated (coated) and communicates at rapid speed. This "upper branch" facilitates heart and breathing rhythm along with innervating the muscles of the soft palate, middle ear, and larynx and pharynx. The chakras that align here are associated with calm and spirituality because the nerves in this area of your body bring your whole system back to balance. When you are feeling safe in your body, you can access your spiritual essence.

What Are Chakras?

Chakras are energy centers that radiate from your inner core. They are felt from the internal layers outward and are distinguished along your skin. You have many energetic tiers in, around, and beyond your body. The chakras have a more condensed flow than the auras. They connect both the internal and external strata of your frame yet extend beyond it. Rest a hand on any energy flow on your body right now. More than likely, you are on or near a chakra.

The seven main chakras are associated with many yogic traditions. In Hatha yoga, the chakras are centering points for meditation. In Kundalini yoga, the kundalini energy in the base of the spine is brought upward through the seven chakras for spiritual awakening. In Kriya yoga, which was taught by Swami Kriyananda and Paramahansa Yogananda, movement techniques are used through the chakras to attain higher spiritual awareness.[36]

Your chakras possess frequencies that match that of the human electromagnetic field.[37] Consider it this way: Your Soul makes up that electromagnetic energy.

How the chakras communicate in trauma processing reflects so much about your human experience. Here is a breakdown of how I see these messages flow.

Body: Root Chakra Reflects Your Human Dimension of Basic Survival

The root chakra energy is located in your pelvic region. It is closest to the earth and represents the energies of human survival. Food and other resources come from the earth. This chakra sits at the lowest branch of the subdiaphragmatic nerve endings. Here the vagus indirectly affects digestive and reproductive jobs. This chakra is reflective of how you move or rest in adulthood. It holds information about how securely your basic needs were met as a child. It may reveal memories related to sexual trauma.

Emotion: Sacral Chakra Reflects Your Patterns of Connecting with Others

The sacral chakra is located in the mid to lower belly, near the belly button. Emotion in this case is connection through patterned behaviors. It represents early energies of your human development. An infant is highly dependent upon a parent to bond with them. Patterns of how you learned to connect are established here. These secure or insecure involvements are felt deeply in the sacral chakra.

---

36. Yoganada, *Autobiography of a Yogi*.
37. Hunt, *Infinite Mind*, 20–21.

Mind: Solar Plexus Chakra Reflects Your Patterns of Self-Identity in a Greater World

The solar plexus is located at the crux of where the two sides of your rib cage meet. After you branch out from family into a larger world, you define your identities among your peers. This meaning is shaped through mind. How deeply you hold on to these identities is felt strongly in the solar plexus chakra. This chakra aligns with the subdiaphragmatic branches of the vagus along the upper digestive tract of the stomach, liver, bile ducts, and adrenal glands—which release cortisol into the system. This is a highly charged energy center that can get more charged when you struggle with identity and connection.

Compassion: Heart Chakra Reflects Your Patterns of Genuine Compassion to Self and Others

The chakras above the diaphragm align with a branch of the vagus that manages your physiological calm and brings you to a loving, safe place with others. This is one of the reasons so many people are drawn to working with the heart chakra. It is a powerful source of healing because the supradiaphragmatic branches connected to the heart and lungs are designed to slow you down. When we slow, we can feel our internal essence. This is why I call this chakra the dimension of compassion.

Connection: Throat Chakra Reflects Your Patterns Through Words and Sound to Establish Connection with Others

The throat chakra makes up a wonderful complexity of vagal fibers that not only allows you to speak but hear. This is the only energy center that manifests sound and becomes the most powerful of all the centers for connection. Sound within a certain range sends signals of safety. If the ranges, called prosody in polyvagal theory, are too high or too low, they register sounds of danger. Sound helps you know if you are safely connected to others.

Spirituality: Third Eye Chakra Reflects Your Comfort with Individual Experiences of Spirituality

The third eye chakra, the dimension of spirituality, brings you inward. Through symbolism and imagery, messages play themselves out here. Ocular nerves in the brain, which send signals to the vagus, facilitate experiences with your internal world. The eyes play a large role in several powerful modalities that work out traumatic energies.[38] The third eye chakra represents the potential for deeper insight, intuition, and higher consciousness as it aligns with the prefrontal cortex of the brain, the area of higher reasoning.

Empathy: Crown Chakra Reflects a Wider Connection Through Empathy

The crown chakra, which I call the dimension of empathy, engages you in an energetically Soulful way. It also seems to circle us right back around to the root chakra to keep this safe human connection going. This chakra sits at the top of your head, between the third and lateral ventricles. This aligns with the thalamus, one of the most important glands in the human body. The thalamus is command central for most sensory nerves and integrates emotional information to the limbic system. Because it contributes to regulation of the safety branch of the vagus nerve, you are able to stay present to others.[39] Allowing someone the space to be heard while you can regulate your own system is at the core of empathy.

---

38. Grand, *Brainspotting*, 69.
39. Porges, *Polyvagal Safety*, 147.

Crystal's Story: A Homecoming

My next client taught me in ways I could never have imagined and
continues to teach me. Through Crystal, I vicariously experienced
what a Soul does when it wants to leave and what reexperiencing
the physical is like when it decides to return.

I was reluctant to take Crystal on. I already had a full schedule,
and I feared my private practice would not be enough for their
needs. Jackie, a friend and former coworker at a local hospital,
called me to refer Crystal. She said her patient was ready to be discharged after being in the intensive care unit for a month following
a brutal knife attack. It was a drug-related crime, and it appeared
Crystal was attempting to buy from a dealer. I didn't know how
stable Crystal would be regarding their addiction since once a week
in a therapist's private practice office usually isn't enough support
for someone who might not be working a recovery program yet.

"Shouldn't they be in treatment first?" I asked my friend on
the phone.

"I know you're busy," she said. "But you're gonna want to work
with this one, C. J. I promise you."

My friend and I have known each other for years, and I also
trusted her professional judgment. "Okay, done."

When Crystal walked into my office a few days later, I was even
more doubtful than ever. It appeared the wounds from the stabbing
were fresh on their throat, and the stiches could be seen above the
collar. A trach tube was still inserted in their neck, and they were
walking with a crutch due to a broken knee from the attack.

I got up to move their seat to a more comfortable position
and helped them sit down. When they glanced up at me, I saw
something reflective in their large brown eyes. It was the look of

someone who had seen things no one else had. That look was profoundly sad, humble, and—joyful. I was intrigued.

I sat across from Crystal to make sure they didn't have to turn their neck. I leaned forward and smiled. "Well, looks like you've had a rough time of it."

Crystal laughed, then gave a soft wheeze. "Yes," they said. "Weirdly, the trouble that I caused for myself was way worse than the pain I was trying to avoid."

Crystal was only twenty-five-years old. A year earlier, their teenage brother died from cancer while on hospice. He had been sick for years. Crystal's father had left the family when they were eight, and their brother was the child from their mother's second marriage. Crystal understood they were non-binary from an early age, but given the chaos in the family over their brother's illness, they never really discussed this with their mother. Crystal and their brother would talk all the time, though. Crystal's stepfather and mother struggled to make ends meet. The stepfather worked two jobs and was barely home. Most of the caregiving fell on Crystal.

The night their brother died, Crystal was in the living room playing video games. When they went into the room to say goodnight, their brother had passed. Crystal could not forgive themselves.

"If only I had been in the room, I could have called 911." They struggled to take in a deep breath. "So, fast-forward," Crystal said, "I started taking his pain pills. It was good for a while, since it really did get rid of a lot of shit I didn't want to feel. However, enough was not enough. I found a pill mill for a while, but that source ran out when the doctor got busted." They shrugged. "So, I found a dealer."

"Is that who beat you up?"

"Yeah, after he realized I was non-binary, he seemed intrigued that I still had"—they raised their hand to make air quotes—"girl parts." They paused. "He raped me and tried to kill me."

I nodded and learned forward a little more to send the signal that I was listening.

"I sort of woke up in the hospital," they said. "Sort of …"

"What do you mean, 'sort of'?" I asked.

They hesitated. "You're cool, right?"

I raised a brow and tried not to smile. "I guess that depends on who you ask."

"I mean, Jackie said you're not gonna doubt my story."

"Try me," I said.

"So." Crystal shifted in their chair and looked uncomfortable. "I wasn't really dead, and when I say I woke up in the hospital, I wasn't really waking up. At least not in the normal sense. I was out of my body during the ambulance ride and then stayed out while I was in surgery."

"Yeah, I hear that happens."

"The part of this that seems so surreal is that I wasn't just watching the doctors work on me. I was talking to"—they paused—"to people. I think behind me."

I nodded. "Do you remember who they were?"

They teared up. "One of them was Jacob, my brother. The others … it was like a wall of them. It was really warm and comforting. I'm calling them a wisdom wall. I couldn't see them, but they were holding me up. But also holding me back from leaving."

"So, it wasn't your time?"

"Yeah." Crystal nodded. "It was like that, but they were also holding me, like I was lying on an incredible bed of light. It was warm and loving, and I didn't want to leave it. Something about lying on that wall was charging me. I could talk to them without words. They were reading my mind, and I was reading theirs."

"That sounds amazing." I smiled. "What were they saying?"

"So much." They shook their head and gazed down at the floor for a few seconds. "So much."

Crystal had an etheric look. I would even say otherworldly. Their frail, pale frame was nearly swallowed up by the dark coat they were wearing. Their hair was nearly white, and you could see where doctors had shaved to stitch their head. My heart burst for the sweet person in front of me. Healing would be a slow journey.

"I didn't feel any of the pain of Jacob's loss when I was on the wall. I felt this calm joy. I would put my hand on the places where the grief had been, and they weren't there. Jacob told me he knew I felt guilty for not being there when he died, but then he said he left exactly because I wasn't in the room, because he couldn't have left if I was there." Crystal teared up. "Because it would have been hard for him to leave me. But he said now I know he will never leave me. He's always here." Crystal looked over at me. "Jacob saw the rape and stabbing. He said he stopped it. He had shouted to a passerby and got into their head enough for them to call the police."

"Wow," I said.

"I didn't know that could be done," Crystal said.

"So, Jacob and that passerby saved your life."

"Yeah, not sure how I feel about that," they joked. "Jacob said he saw the grief pain on my body before the rape. He could see the dark colors around me like bruises. They floated in and out of me. That's what it felt like—like my Soul and body had been bruised by losing my baby brother. That pain was just too much."

I very seldom tear up in a session, but I could feel my eyes welling. I nodded, worried my voice would crack.

Crystal went on. "He said he understood why I was using. There was no judgment, no shame. He just understood. The wisdom wall did too." They breathed in. "I used to miss him so much. Now"—they shook their head—"now, I talk to him all the time, and I swear I hear him respond in my head. He's not gone; I just can't physically hold him anymore."

I smiled and nodded.

"The wisdom wall showed me things about myself that I didn't know," Crystal said. "It was like they were saying leaving this life now wasn't part of my chosen path. I didn't like that. I was watching the doctors stitching up my body and seeing how distorted it looked. I didn't want to go back down there. They understood. They were letting me hang in this light. I kinda joked that they were like the charger, and I was the phone.

"I kept looking down at that body and remembered the emotional pain I felt in it. I wasn't in pain in the wall. Then I realized I was gonna feel a whole new level of pain from broken bones if I went back. If I could feel that much emotional pain in my body, I was scared to feel that level of physical pain."

"That makes sense," I said.

"What if I started using again? If I stayed on the wisdom wall, I wouldn't have to feel the rape pain either."

I nodded.

"I could see the energies of that trauma floating around the lump of flesh that was me." Crystal looked up to see if I was still listening. "That body was experiencing these things even though I wasn't in it. It was so weird. I could see pain from the physical hurt, but that body felt pain from the trauma of it all."

I nodded. "Wow."

"I stayed on the wall for a long time, but somehow the body wasn't dead," they said. "I saw my parents in the waiting room.

My mom looked terrified and defeated. I suddenly realized that I had been so absorbed in my own grief that I really hadn't paid attention to hers. I mean, Jacob was her son. I suddenly deeply understood how she was feeling in a way I could not before. She was gonna lose her other kid. She couldn't lose us both."

I smiled as Crystal looked up at me.

"I don't actually remember how I got back in," they said. "I did wake up in the hospital room after the surgery. That's when I met your friend Jackie. She told me she was a victims' advocate and wanted to help me." Crystal smiled. "So, there. I don't care if you think I'm crazy. I know what I know and that has changed everything."

"Well." I smiled, then drew in a deep breath. "I think, if you choose to work with me, I'm gonna be learning more from you than you will from me."

They nodded. "Cool."

I honestly didn't know how to conceptualize my approach for Crystal, but I started where I like to start with everyone, collaborating on what they want from our work and discussing how they imagine they will be as the work progresses. Both of us understood that Crystal was going to have to adjust to being in their body again. For me, I had no idea what that would look like. That is where they had to take the lead. They experienced facets of their physical form that most of us will never comprehend.

Crystal and I discussed doing weekly sessions to start. Given their mother had to still drive Crystal to my office, we discussed doing a hybrid of telehealth and in-person sessions. The second week of working together, we were online.

"We physically hurt," they said, "but not to the level we thought we would. The doctor seems surprised at how rapidly my wounds are healing. We told her about my experience. She joked that maybe this wisdom wall was like a rapid-growth fertilizer, that I have more of something in me now that is stronger healing."

I laughed.

"Regardless," Crystal said, "I'm just happy that everyone helping me is cool when I tell them about my wall." They pulled their collar down. "Look."

"What the—?"

The stiches were out, and there was little more than a slightly purple line across their neck.

"That's amazing. I don't know what to say. How are you sleeping?" I was listening for signs of flashbacks that can appear in sleep.

"Other than a few achy moments, really well."

"So," I said, "maybe the way for me to ask this question is: How do you feel different in your body these days versus before the rape?"

They thought for a long while.

"In some ways we don't feel the same, but that has so much to do with knowing what life is now." They shook their head. "Paying attention to the body is interesting. My heart beats slower because I can calm more easily. What did you say that was?"

"Vagal tone."

"The body is tired and sleeping a lot, but there is great joy inside."

I wondered if Crystal would ever need to process any trauma, as I have never worked with someone with such a profound near-death experience. Maybe having such a strong connection to their spiritual force was shifting everything in their body in ways there was no reference for.

Our sessions became more about working through the experiences of before and after the near-death experience and how this could help make new meaning in their life. Crystal reported no desire to use drugs. Even though they were in a mandated drug testing program, they did this with an understanding it would be cleaning up the old part of their life. Crystal is my unfinished story. We have been working for a while on helping them decide how they want to use this experience to heal others. They returned to college and started a pre-law degree.

"I want to become a victims' advocate," they said. "I think this is where I want to go with this."

The Three Vagal Pathways You Are Always Traveling

Not so long ago, the medical community believed you had only two neural pathways of importance—the sympathetic and parasympathetic branches—that managed arousal or calm in your nervous system. It was conceptualized that the sympathetic branch activated to respond to threats. It was also posited the parasympathetic branch brought you to calm, acting like an on-off switch. This approach did not explain the many complexities of our human responses.[40]

In the early 1990s, a researcher in psychophysiology named Dr. Stephen Porges put forth a new theory; it was called polyvagal theory. He proposed that the vagus nerve serves many and varied purposes beyond bodily functions. He discussed how the vagus makes up our physiological, behavioral, and emotional states and is a huge component in how we can find safe connection with others. His approach has helped honor so many individuals who have struggled with feeling they were "overreacting" to situations or being "too emotional" or defensive, perhaps due to early childhood maltreatment and an inability to feel safety in certain

---

40. Ogden, Minton, and Pain, *Trauma and the Body*, 29.

circumstances. Polyvagal theory now helps us to understand many of these reactions are neurobiological states programmed into a person's nervous system based on perceived threatening experiences in their past. Polyvagal theory gives people the power to access healing without the shame that they are "too intense."

This heavy-lifting nerve is also the conduit for your humanity. It is at once your spiritual connector to your inner knowing and your gauge of the outside world, facilitating opportunities for loving bonds with others and sending messages to run, hide, or freeze if you are in trouble. Thanks to the vagus, you can smile, laugh, cry, and speak—all social signals that let people know you are emotionally available (or not). Your neurobiology assists in helping you assemble in groups, sit quietly and breathe, or move in playful joy. Your vagus scans for you. Over your lifetime, with the help of the brain, it has stored memories of times, places, and people when you were both safe and unsafe.

The vagus nerve has three pathways, which we can also call complexes. These complexes register states of awareness. These states are safety, mobilization, and immobilization. These pathways are neither good nor bad. For instance, some people think mobilization only puts you in a state of fight-or-flight response, but we mobilize in play, exercise, and basic everyday movements as well. Like the brake, accelerator, and transmission in your car that get you to stop, go, or slow, these complexes help you manage how to be in your daily life, and they are always working for you. They are not static one-then-the-other states. You can be calm and play with someone, which activates safety and mobility states. You can be immobile and safe after sex. These vagal states combine, ebb, flow, and change. They are always shifting and subtly "reading the room" for you, many times before you are even aware they are doing it.

How well your vagus reads that room has much to do with its health, called vagal tone. The health of the vagus is not just about nutrition and exercise. You most definitely need to care for your nervous system in this way. However, just like the tone of your muscles, which indicates how well you maneuver everyday motions, vagal tone is an indicator of how easily your nervous system manages stressors and regains a sense of safety. Does your heart return to a normal rate following a stressful event? When you are in a safe situation, does your body experience calm or does it continue to read signs of unrest? How regular is your digestion? How deeply does anxiety rule the day for you? How often do you feel yourself shutting down even when you don't want to?

Like the engine in your car, you cannot see its condition unless you are regularly checking under the hood. However, if the car hesitates, stalls, overheats, or turns off when you are driving, you know it's time for some servicing. Become aware of how your body feels in various situations. Be curious and open and you will notice the shifts and energy movement. Don't judge the experiences since that is one sure way to get overly stimulated. Just notice the sensations and breathe. In this way, you are paying attention to what's under the hood.

Neuroception

A term that Porges developed is *neuroception*.[41] Neuroception is how these vagal pathways construe situations before you're even aware of what is happening. In some cases, this might feel like a sixth sense. For instance, you just know that person you met is lying to you or that street you are about to walk down doesn't

---

41. Porges, *Polyvagal Safety*, 82,

feel right. You can't say why, but you feel it in your "gut." Physical responses of neuroception may be eyes blinking or shoulders jerking at a noise. Babies cry when they are startled. People freeze when they are scared.

Neuroception can be difficult if you have suffered traumatic events, especially when your body and mind were developing in childhood. This is because your nervous system is now working overtime to protect you against threats that may or may not be there. Your system can register a hyper- or hypo-arousal to a place, smell, face, or sound that holds upsetting memories. You may realize this reaction does not fit the current situation, but somehow your body still does what it does. This is referred to as *faulty neuroception*.[42]

Using the car metaphor, faulty neuroception misreads directions because the GPS is not properly working. The directions are misleading you. The question is: How can you become more aware of faulty neuroception? The first step to healing psychologically and physically is knowing where the struggle lies. Your body will tell you. In fact, your body has been needing you to listen for a while. It is not a troublesome child wanting to act up if you let it; your body is a scared child asking to be heard.

Some questions you can answer for yourself are:

- What places or situations bring back distressing memories?
- How does my body respond when I am near that place?
- What people hurt me in my past?
- How does my body respond when I think of them?

---

42. Porges and Porges, *Our Polyvagal World*, 25.

If answering any of these questions generates strong responses (either overstimulation or understimulation), remember the breathing techniques from chapter 1. This will help instill well-being into your body. When you distinguish your body's messages, you have a better chance of not getting stuck in ruts as you travel your life journey. When you can do this, your GPS becomes more effective and can move you forward.

So, let's explore in more detail your three neurobiological states based on polyvagal theory.

Traveling the First Pathway: Safety

The vagus nerve pathway that calms and instills a sense of safety in your body is called the ventral vagal complex. It is part of the parasympathetic branch that fosters connection. This branch directs signals to the brain that you are okay. Those signals assist in lowering your heart rate and blood pressure. Your muscles relax. You can take deeper breaths. Your digestion returns to normal. Even your voice softens and your attention shifts as you are able to be more present and safer for others.[43] This is the branch that communicates rapidly because it is myelinated. Myelination means the nerves are insulated with a fatty sheath that helps transmit information along your heart, lungs, throat, and ears faster.

The quicker you can return to a state of safety after an upset, the more resilient your nervous system is. Techniques such as breathing, moving, or seeking safe places with kind people help. This is called down-regulating. When you make efforts to soothe yourself in this way, it is like tapping the car brake so you have more control over how fast you are going. Engaging the ventral

---

43. Schwartz, *Applied Polyvagal Therapy in Yoga*, 21.

vagal complex to calm is referred to in polyvagal terms as the vagal brake.

When your safety pathways are engaged, your ability to stay present with others increases. Through smiles and soft tones in your voice you can resume chatting and laughing with someone. Even your inner ear muscles shift so you hear the people around you more clearly. These nerve fibers, with the help of other sensory nerves in the brain, help you gauge the social cues of others.

Safety is often thought of as only physical. However, safety includes emotional, psychological, and even financial well-being. Limited resources or social marginalization contribute to a sense of uncertainty. People who manipulate or gossip or lie purposefully instill fear. In supportive communities, people are accepting of you, and in this case, humans are safer in numbers.[44] However, if there are no safe people in your life to connect with, regulating your system by spending time with pets, listening to music, engaging in movement, or going on walks in nature can instill calm.

EXERCISE
Writing Prompt: Safety

This exercise is an attempt to help you define concepts of safety that can be felt but sometimes not seen.

- What does safety mean to you?
- In what environments do you feel safest?
- What does safety feel like in your body?
- With whom do you feel safe?
- What about these people makes you feel safe?

---

44. Porges, *The Polyvagal Theory*, 32.

- Are there times of the day, month, or year when you feel safest? Why?
- What are the times of the year that you feel least safe? Why?

Now that you have defined some places and faces that are safe and how this feels, let's further explore how the ventral vagal complex works for you.

★ ★ ★

Activating the ventral vagal complex isn't just about total relaxation. This branch of your system is vital in unsafe or perceived unsafe situations. When you face scary situations, you need to stay aware. The ventral vagal complex can keep you engaged as other branches of your vagus nerve are in a heightened state. For instance, you might want to run, fight, or shut down when your math teacher discusses you're about to fail the class, but that would make things worse. So, you breath, notice your racing heart and dry mouth, but maintain enough presence to discuss what your options can be.

In Fear: Ventral vagal activity keeps you present and helps you to interpret a person's body language. Are they looking you in the eye or is their gaze shifting to other things? Are they glaring? How are they sitting or standing? What is the tone of their voice? Despite seeking information outside of you to determine if you are safe, listen internally; your body won't lie.

In Joy: Ventral vagal activity allows your system to calm by slowing your heart rate and breathing. Oxytocin, that neuropeptide that plays such a strong role in social bonding, increases and a warmth may spread across your heart and your stomach.[45] It is peaceful. You may feel the urge to sing or laugh, as your throat is not constricted. All is well when you are safe with others and in places that create calm.

Imagine you laughing with those you love and have known for years. You are calm and safe.

Traveling the Second Pathway: Mobilization

Mobilization comes from the sympathetic branch of the vagus nerve. It's what we would consider the fight-or-flight response to a threatening situation. In threat, mobilization provides your body with a cortisol release from your adrenal glands and injects this hormone into your system. It prepares you to act. Cortisol tells your heart rate to increase, your muscles to tense, and your breathing to shorten. When you perceive a lack of safety, your brain floods messages and memories to the nervous system. The brain operates on the lower tiers that relate more to emotion or physical reactions when you are under duress.

The sympathetic branch engages as we go about our day with regular activities. The healthiest thing you can do for yourself when you are feeling activated and the threat is minimal is to walk it out. Move, stretch, or even hum. That is what our bodies are designed to do.

This next writing prompt will help you define times you have experienced sympathetic engagement.

---

45. Schwartz and Mailberger, *EMDR Therapy and Somatic Psychology*, 21.

EXERCISE
Writing Prompt: Mobilization

- Do you remember an event when you didn't feel safe? What did you experience in your body? Where did you feel this?
- What does your body feel like when you are stuck in rush hour traffic? What is your perception when you are in traffic?
- What did you think about your response after you down regulated?
- Are there times you have gotten up to move because you did not feel safe even though you realized later there was no threat?
- Think of a time you were active and happy. What were you doing? Who were you with? Where do you feel that in your body?

Now that you have defined movements that felt safe and unsafe, let's further explore how the sympathetic complex works for you.

★ ★ ★

Sometimes we act when there is no threat because our nervous system engaged to keep us safe. That happens when situations or people in our past hurt us and our system is now conditioned to respond at all costs.

In Fear: There are times we think we would react one way during scary circumstances, yet we respond completely different. This is how our neuroception works. It can override our beliefs about ourselves and what we think we might do.

If you are surprised by some responses you have had in the past, don't be hard on yourself. When an event happens, your mind usually doesn't have time to think it through. It is your nervous system that does the job in the moment. If you don't respond in the way you thought, this is not a character flaw.

In Joy: Mobilization also helps you connect with others. This is what children do every day. They jump, skip, and run as ways of connecting. How do you feel after a walk, run, or exercise class? If you are doing this with friends, it feels really good during and after, doesn't it? You've moved and coregulated with laughter and conversation in a shared experience.

Getting going is a natural state and is important to access. If you are under no threat but have perceived a threat (like anxiety), you need to move and not shut down. Lack of movement, especially in the upper regions of your body where you can access ventral vagal energy, is a contributor to depression. If my clients are starting to feel pulled-down emotionally, I have them stretch their arms, neck, and shoulders. Upregulating in these cases is a great thing, and you can do it for yourself. Even gentle stretching can change your mindset. What is the saying? "Move it or lose it"?

Traveling the Third Pathway: Immobilization

The freeze response comes from the dorsal vagal complex of the vagus nerve. This is the pathway that can immobilize you in times of danger. This might look anything like fainting to not being able to get off the couch. When this freeze response overtakes the system, you might even lose control of your bowels or bladder since this complex contributes to digestion. It can override your voluntary control of bodily functions. Dorsal vagal activation conserves energy during periods of prolonged intensity.

Many times this freeze response can be interpreted as fatigue or depression. It contributes to dissociation, which takes you temporarily out of your body. Getting back into connection with your body will eventually regulate you, but this might be a while. I have discussed this with clients who have early childhood medical or sexual trauma. Immobility and dissociating from their body was the way they survived. So, they find themselves easily dissociating as adults.

To come back from such states requires working through the branches of your nervous system like a ladder.[46] Moving from immobility requires making your way to mobility before you can get to safety.

Sometimes this needs to be as simple as imagining yourself moving first, then slowly physically moving. Breathing brings you back, so does humming, moving facial features (try forcing a smile and notice how that feels), and slowly turning your head.

---

46. Dana, *The Polyvagal Theory in Therapy*, 9.

EXERCISE
Writing Prompt: Immobilization

- Was there a time when something unsafe happened and you didn't move?
- Did you wish you could have fought or ran?
- Did you think you chose to be still?
- What did you tell yourself about being still after the danger passed?
- Did you judge yourself or tell yourself that you must have wanted something to happen?
- Did that immobilization create a sense that you were not in your body?
- Do you remember what that experience of not being in your body was like?
- Now that you know being still was your nervous system's way of keeping you safe, can you be kinder to yourself?

Now that you have defined immobilization that feels safe and unsafe, let's further explore how the dorsal complex works for you.

* * *

In Fear: Once your system has immobilized, it is vital to understand what is happening. This empowers you with awareness. When you are present to what is occurring, you possess equilibrium. This will guide you out of a dorsal vagal state even as you are experiencing one.

Be aware of your breath. If you are not breathing deeply, pull a few breaths into your belly. At the very least, fill your lungs. Judging this state is the last thing you should do. Just notice. By observing, you are bringing control back into your situation.

In Joy: A powerful description of how you can experience an immobilized response is after an orgasm. The body responds in safety but is temporarily frozen. If you are feeling safe with your partner, this state of both safety and immobilization is pleasant. Another example might be when you are laying on the couch cuddling with your pet or a loved one. There are many times dorsal vagal activation can bring you into peaceful experiences that don't dissociate you. This branch helps regulate your body's digestion. It slows the heart rate and increases secretion of digestive enzymes. In this way, the body is conserving energy by relaxation.

Observe your system. How can you be empowered to shift states? Being curious, even in the midst of a chaotic or stressful moment, can keep you attuned. Opening to the warmth of a loving hug, laugher, or smile feels very present in your body.

EXERCISE
Making Way for the Angel Within

In my early years as a therapist, I was shown that people struggling with depression cave forward as a protective measure. This was before I had become polyvagal informed in my practice, but it was certainly an accurate insight. That awareness helped me to assist people who were struggling. I found some wonderful stretches and exercises to engage and activate what I now know to be the ventral vagal complex.

When we slump forward, we protect those very tender communication devices that emanate from our vagus nerve and organs. We are closing off chakric energy. Our face is no longer available to people. We have shut down to connection. Pulling in the chest cavity closes off important organs and nerves and cuts off their literal breathing room.

Creating space in your chest cavity reclaims enjoyment. You don't have to be depressed to slump. Most of our daily life is centered around a computer, electronic device, or a desk. The question is, does the slumping affect your mood and ability to connect to others?

Here are two very active exercises that help support your shoulders and back by using a wall. These exercises will increase responsiveness of the ventral vagal complex and engage mobility in the sympathetic branch. I am calling these guardian angel exercises because, well, we have many guardians that watch over us along this journey.

I have set these up so you can use a wall as a stabilizer. The wall will also help you increase neck alignment since tightened vertebrae contribute to pinched and malfunctioning cranial nerves. Aligning your back and neck with the assistance of the wall also slows blood flood to the brain as it affects the vertebral arteries.

Guardian Angel Stretch

Examine the following diagram and know your limits if you have shoulder or neck issues. Your back should be flat against the wall with feet about a foot from it to stabilize. That includes shoulders and arms as well as your head. Chin should not be turned down but straight. Don't wear socks if you have hardwood floors, as your feet might slip. Examine the posture to make sure you can do this.

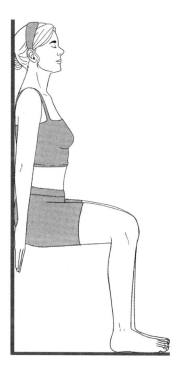

Figure 4: Guardian Angel Pose

Guardian Angel Wings

Once you are stable, turn your palms outward. Then, as if you were making angels in the snow, slowly slide your outstretched arms along the wall. Reach up and keep your arms over your head a moment. Then slowly slide your arms back down to your sides. Repeat.

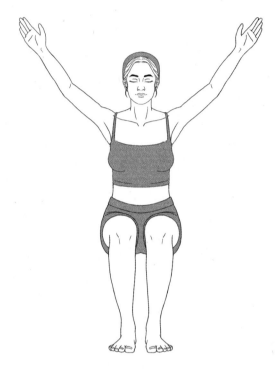

Figure 5: Guardian Angel Wings

Guardian Angel Wings (Modified)

This modification of the previous exercise helps anyone with shoulder issues by keeping the arms bent. With the same placement against the wall, including your head, bend your arms with palms facing out and slide your arms up and down. You are still making angels—just with arms bent. Do this as many times as you wish.

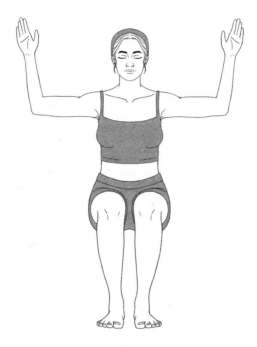

Figure 6: Guardian Angel Wings (Modified)

Once you are done, slide your heels back to the wall. This way you can push yourself up with stabilization. Stand straight. Take a deep diaphragmatic breath. Notice how your body feels. Has this elevated your mood? Where does your energy flow?

Summary

The vagus nerve is the longest branch in your autonomic nervous system, which is part of your central nervous system. Autonomic means automatic, as your lungs, heart, and digestive organs are automatically working in the background. While the vagus nerve is bilateral in nature, just like your brain, it has three pathways within it that register states of safety. These states are important as they define how you are identifying your connection in the world and with others. These pathways are safety, mobilization, and immobilization. While these pathways are distinct, they work in tandem and are always gauging for you.

Understanding when you are experiencing these states is powerful. *Neuroception* is a term devised by Porges, who developed polyvagal theory. Neuroception is how these vagal pathways construe situations before you're even aware of what is happening.

Chakras are energy centers that radiate from your inner core. Your body has possibly hundreds of them, as they seem to be energetic flow centered around your nerve fibers. The seven main chakras discussed in this book are associated with many yogic traditions, including Hatha, Kundalini, and Kriya yoga. These seven energy centers seem to possess psychological dimensions that represent your human experience. In this book, I discuss them as dimension of your body (survival) through the root chakra; dimension of emotion (attachment patterns) through the sacral chakra; dimension of mind (identity) through the solar plexus; dimension of compassion (safety) through the heart chakra; dimension of connection (tones) through the throat chakra; dimension of spirituality (imaginal) through your third eye; and dimension of empathy (connected awareness) through the crown chakra.

How the chakras communicate in trauma processing reflects so much about your human experience. Your personal awareness and internalized past are expressed through these energy centers. Applying a curious approach to what your body is experiencing is a way forward.

CHAPTER 3
YOUR EARTHLY JOURNEY

⎯⎯⎯●⎯⎯⎯⎯⎯●⎯⎯⎯

Let's start your journey by engaging more deeply with your lower body, where the essential chakras of body, emotion, and mind work hard for you. Those subdiaphragmatic branches of your vagus nerve are also constantly communicating. The way I encourage you to engage with this area of your body is through grounding, preferably with natural surroundings. If you can gain confidence in your physical self, you can reconnect to your body in a way that restores access to your inner light. If you have disconnected from your body and see it as an adversary, then I hope you will learn to befriend it again.

Feeling secure in your body is the first leg of your journey. That vehicle gets you where you want to go. Your body is the access to your innermost cave, the deep forest that eventually leads to your Soul. These pathways may be mildly familiar, but due to very little foot traffic, it is not clear what route to take.

In this unexplored space, the ground is slippery and dank from the overflowing rocky streams that cut into the earth. The sun is an unreliable visitor here. The scents are visceral and enveloping. It is primeval, yet when you rest within it, there is something magical about this place. These woods, inhabited with ancient trees, uneven terrain, and unidentified species of plants, feel consecrated. This hallowed ground conjures both fear and awe in the core of you. Hoots echo. Winged creatures flutter and call into a distance that is hidden. You can feel the eyes of animals, perhaps dead and alive, that watch your presence as you amble through. They guard this place. They are as curious and uncertain as you are. That human tension of body, mind, and Soul is felt here. While your mind fears any experience it cannot understand, your body—because it is driven by Soul—anticipates the next bend in the path.

Grounding the Essential Chakras

One of the important pieces of knowledge we are taught as trauma therapists is to help a client manage their affect tolerance. As I have been stating, affect is a direct result of responses stored in your brain and nervous system. When you understand these are sensations programmed into your "wiring" based on past experiences, you can slow your body down, or galvanize it back to present awareness. Managing your nervous system gives you a chance to ultimately reach that softer core of emotion.

Affective responses are strongly felt within the gut region. Not to say that you don't feel intensity to perceived threat in other parts of your body, but that belly can be a doozy sometimes. Implicit memory, which is memory that is felt but not easily pulled to mind, shows up here. Heed these messages using the breathing techniques I introduced to you in chapter 1. Befriend them.

The chakras in this region are:

- The root chakra, which encompasses the body's experiences.
- The sacral chakra, which encompasses the childhood attachment experiences.
- The solar plexus, which encompasses aspects of your identities in the outside world.

The energy centers of these lower chakras store felt memories from prebirth into older childhood. It is this physical terrain that is asking for the most care and healing. If you listen to these messages in the same way you would young children asking to be heard, you can approach that visceral discomfort that shows up here with less fear or shame.[47] When they are not responded to, children tend to get louder. If they are heard, they calm. If they aren't, they eventually give up and shut down—not unlike your body.

Since the abdomen and digestive tract get tricky with how they signal emotional distress, you may have detached from them. If your autonomic nervous system learned to release bodily waste at the first sign of danger, fear of intense "emotions" became a regular pattern. Any potential stomachache could be an embarrassment and lead you right into the bathroom stall in a public place (remember our discussion about the immobility state of the dorsal vagal branch). The more messages of safety you can reprogram into your body, the less likely this will happen over time. When you learn how to revisit and hold space for what your body is trying to tell you, giving it love and kindness, life changes.

Body: The Root Chakra

Root chakra energy is aligned with the lower intestines and sex organs. This is the region of sexual responses, birth, and elimination of food waste, which are some of the most rudimentary human functions you have.

The vagus nerve plays a direct and indirect role in this area, as it sends signals to other autonomic branches in the lumbar and pelvic regions. During childbirth, the vagus influences the release

---

47. Sweezy, *Internal Family Systems Therapy for Shame and Guilt*, 117.

of oxytocin. This hormone stimulates uterine contractions and helps the cervix to dilate. This area of your body is the base of the hypothalamic-gonadal axis that ends in either the ovaries or the testes, which the vagus plays a role in managing.

When this area of your body has been sexually violated, it contains unprocessed memories of the trauma through the skin and organs. The nervous system registers threat and dysregulates. Many people become immobile and disconnect from their pelvic region or that dysregulation might manifest as impulsive or compulsive behaviors and hypersexuality.[48] Trauma to this region of the body can also happen during surgery, complicated childbirth, a car accident, or a number of other experiences. You are the only one who can discern your history and how the energy in that region of your body feels.

Physically, if you are unbalanced in the pelvic region, there is imbalance all the way up your shoulders, neck, jaw, and head. Your torso alignment affects the configuration of your spine, which affects your nervous system. Physical misalignments reveal themselves in the less dense energy of your chakras. Physical therapists that specialize in pelvic health can restore your body's alignment for greater ease and connection. They can introduce you to how to rebalance in your pelvic floor, pelvic diaphragm, ligaments, and muscles.[49] Your energy centers will naturally flow as a result. Regaining connection and balance in the pelvic region is reclaiming connection to your root chakra energy.

Creating safety in this region of your body using both the mobility and the immobility branches of the vagus nerve can be done through rest and fun, playful, and joyful movement. Yoga,

---

48. Ogden, Minton, and Pain, *Trauma and the Body*, 39.
49. Stein, *Heal Pelvic Pain*, 10.

the natural movement of walking, and intuitive stretching are helpful. Through a polyvagal perspective, moving in ways that feel right and safe for you are primary. Children connect through play and laughter.[50] So can you.

Just being outside in fresh air and sunshine can also bring safety to your body. Through the earth, all your physical needs are met. Plants provide food. Water and air help you to survive. Soil, sand, and greenery connect to you as much as you connect to them. You don't have to define yourself as an outdoorsy person to know the benefits of sunshine on your face or cool grass beneath your feet. No special hiking gear or camping equipment has to be purchased. Your body needs to connect to the soil it has been designed to traverse. A process called earthing proves this.[51]

Earthing

Earthing is a term used to describe ways to regulate your body by connecting to the earth. Direct contact with the ground elevates mood, helps you sleep, and improves heart health.[52] Scientists are learning that disconnecting from nature, with regular exposure to blue light and radio frequency waves from electronic devices, creates an imbalance and negatively affects your health.[53] The longer you stay away from those screens, the less absorption rate of radio frequencies your body has.

---

50. Porges, *Polyvagal Safety*, 192.
51. Ober, Sinatra, and Zuker, *Earthing*.
52. Chevalier and Sinatra, "Emotional Stress, Heart Rate Variability, Grounding, and Improved Autonomic Tone," 154–60.
53. Oschman, Chevalier, and Brown, "The Effects of Grounding (Earthing) on Inflammation, the Immune Response, Wound Healing, and Prevention and Treatment of Chronic Inflammatroy and Autoimmune Diseases."

Studies show that the earth has a vast supply of electrons. Electrons from the earth transport energy chains into your mitochondria. The mitochondria are organized structures within cells that have many functions for the life of a cell. One of mitochondria's primary jobs is to generate a chemical energy called adenosine triphosphate (ATP). ATP is the main chemical energy source in a cell. ATP is used by all types of cells, from bacterial to human cells; it's a life force. If you remember that your embodied Soul is a bioelectrical being, it makes sense that all aspects of you are elevated when you connect to nature.

A barefoot day at the beach or taking your shoes off at the park charges the potentially 200,000 nerves that end in your feet. The nerves traverse from the sciatica and lower spine and begin a dialogue of sensory experiences throughout the body. Whether or not you are attuning to this energetic flow, it is there. Your vagus and the highway of nerves that communicate with your organs thank you.

Along the nerve centers in your feet, there are chakras located in the middle of the arches. They are naturally connected to the root chakra as energy runs up your legs. When your feet are planted, a floodgate of electrons rush along the channels of your legs. They work upward. Spend time barefoot on cool soil, and you will feel the activation.

Given your body is made mostly of water, it also acts as a conductor for these electrons. If you think in terms of calming the nervous system, then you can see these electrons are also cleansing toxins—seen and unseen—that have been circulating in your body. Inflammation then calms as your cortisol regulates.

The following exercise shares ways to connect. Notice how you feel afterward.

EXERCISE
Earthing Ideas

If you are housebound, there are several products that state they will produce similar grounding effects on your body as being in the outdoors will. These are mats for sleeping, patches on your skin that attach to rods outside your home, and jewelry made with conducting materials. There are even grounding mats for your office chair. Spend time researching any of these.

However, if you are not housebound, just going outside will be your least expensive and most immediate source of relief. Just be consistent and intentional with connecting. Listen to your body. Breathe.

Here are some simple suggestions for how to ground to the earth:

- Hug a tree with bare feet firmly on the roots or ground.
- Find a patch of grass to sit or stand barefoot on.
- Picnic in the park.
- Walk on the beach.
- Sit by a stream and place hands and feet on rocks.
- Garden with bare hands and feet (potted plants as well).
- Soak feet in river or stream.
- Do yoga outside.
- Intuitively move on grass.
- Walk anywhere soft without shoes.
- Nap on the ground.

Walking outside engages your leg muscles, glutes, hips, and lower back, which increases energy flow through the root, sacral, and solar plexus chakras. Movement through walking is what your body was designed for. Yet, we get just as disconnected from our walking as we do from the ground itself. Are you checking your phone or talking on the phone when you walk?

As you age, your legs and the lower portion of the body get used less. Physicians state that inflammation in the body can generally begin in the feet. Aging affects balance and coordination due to changes in the nervous system and proprioception (how your muscles sense movement and action). A sedentary life leads to inflammation. If you have spent a lifetime dissociating from your physical self, possibly through food, substances, or lack of movement, reconnecting is vital.

Bring those muscles back to life. They get you moving toward the places you want to go and help you leave places you don't want to be. Movement *is* grounding. It is the grown-up version of play if we let it be. Stay connected. As you connect with movement you are naturally engaging with your etheric energies as well. You don't have to think too hard to do this. Your body is designed to flow. Let it.

The following is a meditation that is intended to help increase chakra energy awareness while standing barefoot on the ground.

EXERCISE
Rooted to the Earth Meditation

The best way to connect to any of the chakra energies in your body is to draw attention to the area through breath. In this exercise, we are going to incorporate the chakras in the feet as well as the root chakra. What a way to optimize your earthing experience. Give yourself time to experience this meditation. There is no hurry. The best thing you can do is ground regularly to the earth. If you struggle with standing, sit on the earth. Rest your palms to the ground. Let your hips feel the connection and stay planted to the ground.

To begin, find an area outside that appeals to you. This can be a garden, lawn, field, beach, hiking path, riverbed, or anything else that draws you. Take your shoes off. Enjoy.

- Stand with feet no more than shoulder width apart. This gives you some balance.
- Spread your toes in a way that lets energy flow but is not too wide.
- Soften your knees but don't feel you have to bend them. They should hold you up but be receptive enough to experience flow.
- Soften the muscles in your arms and shoulders to release tension.
- Look straight ahead, as this will balance your body.
- Take a look around and remind yourself that you are safe.
- Sway back and forth slightly for a few seconds. This helps you find your center and settles your feet into the ground.
- Pull a breath into your pelvic region by softening your belly.
- Notice how long you can leave the breath there before you need to slowly exhale.
- Notice your feet, legs, and pelvis without judgment.
- Breathe in a flow that is natural to you.

- Attune to the temperature of the earth. Is it warm or cool?
- Just be with the experience.
- Notice the natural scents around you.
- Are you feeling tightness or calm?
- Where does the energy flow?
- Continue to slowly pull your breath into the pelvic region.
- Don't force a flow. Whatever the experience is, that is right for you.
- If negative thoughts about your body rise up, just let them hang gently outside of you.
- Breathe and notice the natural scents around you.
- Is there a breeze? Sunshine?
- What is the temperature of the air?
- Breathe deeper into your hips and lower belly.
- Thank this area for all the work it has done through the years.
- Just be.

Once you are done with the above meditation, stretch and move your legs in a way that feels right for you. What do you notice?

Remember that connection to your body is vital for your spiritual journey. Your body is not a hinderance to your Soul. Body is the vehicle your Soul drives along your life path. There is no duality. Body is not bad, and Soul is not good. While you are here, this is a collaboration. You are a Soul inhabiting human form. Your job is to help increase the mastery of steering it.

★ ★ ★

Souls understand that love is the only force in the universe. Within you is great love, though down here we get disconnected and turned around from that truth. We experience pain and disconnection from loved ones who also got turned around. We act out that illusion of disconnection and struggle to find a way back to connection. Sometimes we think that if we just try harder to engage in a spiritual training, we will reclaim the love we lost. We have to be careful that perfection of a spiritual practice does not get prioritized over simple acts of self-love and kindness.

The story of my next client is a moving example of how a person can restrict their body and rigidly employ a spiritual practice until it makes them sick—just to be loved. My client saw everything in either-or terms. She was either spiritual or she was nothing. The body was an obstacle to getting love. Her duality was killing her.

Anna's Story: Restriction and the Lotus

Anna came to residential treatment because of her addiction to amphetamines. To avoid depression and feelings of inadequacy, Anna was constantly seeking the high of stimulants. She was forty pounds thinner than her healthy weight. At thirty years old, she had already suffered one stroke, and her heart was weak. The amphetamines were also her way to restrict food. She was terrified she would gain weight now that she was in a treatment center and not using stimulants.

Anna had harsh parents who were always pushing her to do better and be something. Her father made regular comments about her appearance. If Anna gained any weight, he would point it out. She had been studying to be a yoga teacher but had been fired by her trainer because Anna wouldn't show up for the classes

she was supposed to teach. Anna insisted she already knew everything she needed to know. She told me the instructor wouldn't listen to her, so she just stopped going.

Each morning in the treatment center, I led mindfulness and
somatic classes for the patients. This was to empower people who
were no longer using their addiction as a defense against the world
to develop some resiliency. Gentle breathing, walking, and attuning in safe ways to their senses were intended to help patients trust
their bodies again.

Anna postured herself as the most knowledgeable person in
the room. She showed up dressed in expensive yoga clothing that
hung off her body because she was so thin. Her use of Sanskrit
terms was flawless regarding yoga poses, or asanas. She would
attempt to take over the class and tell others they were doing things
wrong—including me.

When the class would perform simple mindfulness breathing,
Anna would fold her legs into a "perfect" lotus position and sit in
the chair with a rigid spine, chin jut forward, palms upward on her
knees. On the surface, Anna looked like a guru. Underneath, she
was straining to hold on to anything that would give her a sense
of identity and power. Now that she had no access to her drug of
choice, she was struggling with how to be in the world.

The clinical team eventually thought it was best that Anna not
attend these mindfulness groups because of the forceful way she
was treating herself (and others who couldn't perform as perfectly
as her). Instead, we brought Anna to art classes and equine therapy. These experiences were out of her comfort zone, and it terrified her. Anna threatened to leave treatment.

With support and individual sessions, Anna began to understand she had various internal resources. She saw how she could

play with color and form in art classes (and get her hands dirty). She slowly began to trust her creativity. She grew comfortable with the horses and was even helping to groom them.

In her individual sessions with me, Anna shared that looking into the eyes of these huge creatures and seeing their gentleness was the first time she felt connected to herself. We broke that down. She started to understand the horses were reflecting a tenderness that she wanted deeply to experience but felt she could not.

"Weird, isn't that?" I said.

Her eyes welled with tears. Anna was starting to access her emotions and trust the flow of them.

Through these new experiences, Anna softened. She opened to her intuition. Her inner world was no longer something she dreaded. Anna saw the many facets of who she was and accepted at times those parts contradicted each other. This allowed her to be more flexible and kinder to herself—and others.

Life became more pleasurable for Anna. She started to comprehend she did not have to be "perfect" to get love. She also understood that her need to be perfect had kept her from showing up to yoga classes because she didn't think she could perform at the ridiculous standard she had set for herself. Even her drug use, she admitted, was a way to combat her impossible expectations.

Anna reached out to her yoga trainer, and they had a long talk. After she left treatment, she started a new kind of yoga practice, one where she and the students could just be. She no longer saw yoga as performative but an opportunity to lovingly engage with her body and emotions.

"When I thought I had to be perfect," she said, "I thought I had to shut out anything in me that didn't look that way. I was crushing my Soul."

Emotion: The Sacral Chakra

Before you entered this world as the person now reading this book, you were a brilliant essence, a Universal Source. That essence took on your current human form. Now that your Universal Essence is inhabiting your body, it works things out through the construct you are living. In this case, construct simply means how your life is shaped. That construct includes the places, experiences and the people you engage with. The ways you love, your desire for affection, and how you relate to people was all shaped very early by family—even before you were born.[54]

How your parents tended to your physical and emotional needs influenced how you tend to yours and others' needs. This emotional map was patterned into your body when you were so young that the only memory you may have is a felt one (implicit). These memories—the pain, the warmth, or the confusion—resonate throughout your whole physical system. From your nervous system's responses to the meaning you make, your patterning plays itself out in the world. This is why I define that sacral chakra as the energy of emotion.

Emotion in this case is the emotion of familiarity. We are all drawn in some hypnotically human way to the familiar. This familiar lies within your nervous system and is revealed (and felt) in the sacral chakra. This dance makes up your interpersonal imprint.[55] If your parents were not affectionate, you may deeply want to hug your children but something keeps you from doing that. If you were told you were worthless, you might have internalized that belief and retreat in shame from new job opportunities. If you were loved and listened to, your body can remain calm during even

54. Bowlby, *Attachment*.
55. Tatkin, *Wired for Love*, 25.

a tense conversation. Those patterns are encoded into your brain and vagus nerve. If you don't know differently, you may tell yourself it is just a character trait.

Some yogi masters have stated the sacral chakra was the chakra involved in the energy of sexual intimacy. Given that attachment theory didn't take hold in Western psychology until the mid-twentieth century,[56] I posit that in this case sexual energy is a lust for the familiar. Emotion regarding this chakra may or may not include the love of your family, but it is certainly founded in the emotional entanglements of your family. We work things out in adulthood that didn't work in childhood through this energy center. Sometimes love is not the same thing as how we connect with intimate partners.

Sacral chakra energy merges with the subdiaphragmatic fibers of the vagus close to the digestive track, intestines, bladder, and lower kidneys. This region is the energy of mother and child through the umbilical cord. At one time, you were one with your mother. The longing for that echoes in your biology.

The neurobiological memories here are strong, and they possess a felt relationship with food. Mothers feed us before we are birthed into a loud, cold world. Our mothers continue to feed us as infants and do so until we can feed ourselves. These layered associations with food as nurturing are complicated and driven by feeling loved and safe—or not. It's a primal combination, this food and loving connection, and it extends out into shared eating experiences in our adult lives. Given this chakra is connected to the organs of digestion, can you see where emotions and food cues become confused?

---

56. Ainsworth, *Patterns of Attachment.*

Alan's Story: Trying to Get to Mom Six Times Over

Alan came to therapy after divorcing his sixth wife. This most recent marriage only lasted eighteen months, and he stated he was the most despondent over this divorce. Alan was a fifty-six-year-old professional who successfully managed a large department in a national corporation. He was educated, well dressed, and disarmingly polite. His politeness seemed to hold up a defense wall against people that kept anyone from accessing his true thoughts and feelings. This made him appear acquiescent and cooperative, but he was unusually stubborn behind it.

"I just don't understand why they leave me," he said within the first several minutes of our intake session. "I give them everything they need. I just ask that they are there for me."

"What does being there for you look like?" I asked.

He shrugged. "You know, they don't work, so I ask for them to prepare dinner and keep up the house. Traditional stuff, I know. Spend time with me. She doesn't need friends if she has me, right?" Then suddenly he burst out crying. "I have reached out to her every day and have asked her not to leave, but she just says she doesn't want to be with me." He held his palm over his belly. "It hurts so much."

Upon further interviewing, it was revealed that this wife was thirty years younger than Alan and that she was caught having an affair with their house painter. Over the course of our history taking, a pattern emerged with the women in his life.

All the women Alan dated and married were underemployed and less educated than him. In two cases, the women were struggling single mothers and gladly latched on to marriage with a successful man. They were also significantly younger than Alan, and as Alan aged, the age gap increased. The womens' ages when they married him ranged from eighteen to twenty-six. The time gap between marriages also was lessening, as this last marriage was only six months in between the previous one.

When we got to the conversation about his early childhood, Alan insisted everything was fine. He was close to his father, who was a retired business executive, and Alan said his father had been a major influence on Alan's own success. He said his mother didn't live with them, but they had a good relationship. As he spoke about his mother, he sat up straighter and rested his hands on his lap. Alan would get avoidant when we would talk about his mother. He would bring the conversation back around to this recent wife, whom he said he loved the most.

At the third session, Alan revealed that his mother abruptly left. Alan was just four years old and an only child. His father, in an effort to look like the good guy (and control his son), told Alan that his mother left because Alan was too troublesome to raise. As he told me this, he broke out into irreconcilable tears again. The four-year-old Alan was aching to be heard.

"Can we just make some space for him?" I said. "Let him in the room a bit."

Alan left a message before his next session that he would need to cancel indefinitely, as his wife wanted to get back with him and everything was good now. I also figured his intense emotional outburst had scared parts of him, as Alan worked so much at managing a composed façade.

Four months later, Alan rescheduled because he was now in the middle of a nasty divorce and felt he needed help.

"I can't help you unless you're open to helping yourself," I said. "How you are going about managing your pain is creating more. Those little children in there are hurting. They are experiencing the trauma of marriage and remarriage. It's too much. They keep reliving their mother's abandonment."

Alan's polite defenses faltered. He looked annoyed. "I am not."

I sat for a moment and let him rant about this divorce and that divorce. Then I asked, "Where are you feeling this intensity in your body?"

He stopped and his eyes widened. "I dunno."

"Can you breathe and just notice what your body is experiencing?"

His expression softened, and he looked like a little boy.

"Regardless of whether or not you want to befriend this intensity in your system, it's already there," I said. "You will just continue to carry it with you."

"I don't want that!"

We began by teaching Alan breathing skills. He even tried some mindful meditation at home. We went slow. The protective parts of him needed to feel competent before he tried something as vulnerable as somatic inquiry.

"I feel like this is the first time in my life I've actually taken a full breath," he said. "I feel a little freer."

Once Alan felt competent with connecting to his body through breath, we explored the energy in his body by just noticing it. Through befriending these energies, he realized he had an access point toward healing.

Alan and his very elaborate ego defense system started trusting me enough to do Internal Family Systems (IFS) processing. It took him some time. Years, in fact. He needed to know that, as a female therapist, I too wouldn't abandon him. Since he had been living a life of female abandonment since he was in preschool, Alan was at once suspicious and overly trusting.

Over time, he was able to reach and heal those young parts that made up his ego defense system. This took intention, compassion for himself, and curiosity. Those ego parts had been wanting to enmesh, control, and even destroy the women in his life to recreate something he never had, which was bonding with his mother and truth from his father.

For two years while we did this therapy, Alan said he didn't want to date. He wanted to know what it was like to genuinely take care of himself and not attempt to regulate others while he was learning to regulate himself. After a while, Alan started dating. He has been with the same woman for several years now. They decided it was healthier for them to show up each day as partners and not lock into a legal document with the illusion no one could ever leave. Alan said he struggles with this sometimes, but he has learned to live in the tension of that.

Minding the Void

If you had a lack of safe connection with your family as a child, then that fear instilled itself deeply within your system. Your belly, the sacral area, feels this. I have seen this during my trauma processing with clients. They sometimes describe it as a "void"—a longing or ache for something in their gut. Sometimes the void reaches all the way down into the root chakra. This void expresses itself in the visceral organs. When you can slow down, breathe, and be with it, the affect doesn't feel so engulfing.

You may never have explicit memories around this deep void. You do, however, feel it. We all do in one way or another. Sometimes the experience of the void comes on swiftly. It is a deep longing, a mysterious desire the brain cannot solve. It gets confused with a need to evacuate the bowels or seek sexual release. Before you even know it, you're up and looking for whatever you think that void wants. In so many cases, the instinct to seek isn't fully conscious. I have had clients report they want to end the sessions so they can eat. They want to go early to their next meeting. Some talk rapidly and sit forward to shift the energy.

For therapists, you can slow this physiological information down for clients and show them how to be curious about the information coming from the body. For other readers, pause a moment and be curious when that sensation rises up. Remind yourself this is just your body asking to be heard. Notice if you have the urge to go do something.

When you were a small child, this affect may have felt engulfing. Awareness is the first part of being mindful of the void so you can bring loving-kindness to it. If the experience is too much, then get up and move. The key is that in a brief moment you were aware of the void. Like some friendships, it may take time to get to know and trust it.

EXERCISE
Emotional Void Breathing

If you struggled with family that did not keep you physically or emotionally safe, this breathing exercise may help. If it is too much and you feel yourself getting under- or overstimulated, then it is a good idea to stop. It may be that a therapist will be more helpful to you; you don't have to travel the healing journey alone.

As always, make sure you are in a safe and sacred space. Breathe using the diaphragmatic breathing you learned earlier. Check in with the lower regions of your abdomen. Rest a hand on your belly in a gentle, loving way.

- Remember a time when you felt a need to eat when you weren't hungry.
- Do not judge that time; just notice what energy arises.
- Be curious about the experience.
- Remember that this memory in your body cannot hurt you.
- Let the energy know you are just here to listen and be interested.
- Befriend this energy and listen to what it has to tell you.
- This may be information, images, color, and archetypes.
- If you feel yourself disconnecting from this energy, just move your toes and remind your body it is safe.
- Let this void know you hear it and honor it.
- Stay with it until the wave fades.
- Notice the urges but don't act.
- Be curious, not judgmental about them.

Depending on what came up, you might want to draw or journal about it. Sometimes deep memories float to the surface that are helpful. An implicit memory of a time we did not get held, fed, tended to, or calmed when we were afraid can still drive us. Yet, we can lean into it and love it as if it was now our own child. It might not make sense to your mind. Let this energy know you are here to help it now. You understand it and will listen.

EXERCISE
Earthing the Sacral Chakra

The following is a meditation that will use earthing techniques to help soothe your sacral chakra energy (and vagus nerve). There are two ways to soothe your nervous system when you feel dysregulated. One is to regulate using many of the exercises I am laying out in this book. Regulation is something you can do for yourself. Coregulation is something two nervous systems can do with each other. You coregulate with your friends, children, pets, and loved ones when you are calm and loving. You can also regulate yourself by coregulating with the earth. So, let's go hug a tree.

- Start by not caring who's watching because who cares what they think.
- Remind yourself that you are safe.
- Reach your arms around the tree you want to hug.
- With bare feet, step on the roots or get as close as you can.
- Connect your belly to the tree.
- Pull a breath into your midsection and let your stomach soften.
- Notice how long you can leave the breath there before you need to slowly exhale.
- Breathe.
- Just be with the experience of your sacral chakra.
- How does this feel in your upper intestinal energy?
- Where does the energy flow?
- Continue to slowly pull your breath into this region.
- Be curious.

- Allow any negative thoughts about this area of your body to float up and linger.
- Let them hang gently outside of you without attaching.
- Breathe.
- Notice the scent of the tree and air.
- Imagine the region of your midsection connecting deep inside of you.
- Imagine the energy of the tree lovingly connecting with you.
- Breathe deeper and let the breath expand anywhere in your body the energy needs to go.
- Thank this tree for all it has done through the years.
- Thank your body for all it has done through the years.
- Just be.

Mind: The Solar Plexus

The solar plexus is the energy of how you see yourself in the outside world. This is identity, and it is a construct of your mind. How you relate to others is part of your own self-rule. Do you control others to feel powerful, or can you stand quietly and confidently in your own energy and leave others to their power?

How identities form is based on childhood experiences. Sometimes those family patterns are clear. Sometimes you might not know what those early dynamics are. Family name, gender identity, what you are called, what you look like, how you relate culturally, or your social skills from childhood get played out in school, then work, socially, and eventually the family you choose. These are learned strategies. The "I do things a certain way because that's what my family did" approach is easy when you first step out into a wider world. It gives you some reference points. I am so-and-so from such-and-such helps you find likeminded community. However, if those learned skills do not blend well with what goes on outside your home, you can struggle to find steady footing.

What about those more subtle ways to relate that were learned? These are how you show affection and emotionally connect. How do you respect others' boundaries? How do you respect your own? How did you learn to gain acceptance from people you love or inspire friends and coworkers to accept you? How do you present to people you socialize with versus people you want to date? How do you act with coworkers versus your boss? Your relationships, whether personal or professional, carry with them the emotional patterns formed by your family. They play out in your nervous system and extended etheric energy.

To some extent we become different people to get different results in various situations. The question is: How deeply do you drift from your authentic truth as you do this?

Who knew that the outside world would ask so much more from you. Who knew the outside world might force you to change old ways that no longer work? Welcome to the energy of the solar plexus. This might be one of the most visceral of the chakras because it carries a heavy—sometimes contrasting—load. The solar plexus energy is on the cusp of what you were and what you can evolve into. This is the tipping point of change.

If you struggle with who you are in your life now, you struggle with feeling safely connected to others. The endocrine system controls when and how your body reacts to stress by releasing cortisol into your system. Uncertainty activates the hypothalamic-pituitary-adrenal axis. You can feel a charge in the stomach and other areas of the digestive tract simply because you're not sure.

As you live a broader life, you are required to stretch and grow. Growth puts you temporarily into uncertainty until you can get new bearings. Where you came from is not necessarily where you are going. We are all asked to do this because this is what your Soul came here to do. You are something greater than what you were.

EXERCISE
Writing Prompt: Noticing Beliefs about Yourself

One of your brain's jobs is to make meaning of all encounters you have as you walk through life because it's trying to form patterns to determine if you are safe. As a result, all of the meaning you possess in your present life is based on past encounters with others. These perceptions could be true—or not.

These journal prompts are meant for some deeper reflection as we all get stuck in assumptions about ourselves. Writing these answers out will help you step back, develop some new perception, and reflect.

Let's explore what you think about yourself:

- In only two sentences, write out who you are.
  - What is the most important aspect of yourself that you want to tell others?
  - Were you surprised by what you wrote? Why?
  - What did you think you would say about yourself?
- How do you engage with others?
  - How do you listen to each family member?
  - What do you think about them?
  - How do you show you care for them?
  - How do you speak to them?
  - How do you listen to casual acquaintances or nonfamily members that you see every day?

- How do you engage with yourself when no one is around?
    - What do you tell yourself?
    - How do those thoughts "feel" in your body?
    - How do you spend time with yourself?

EXERCISE
Writing Prompt: Noticing Beliefs about How Others Perceive You

Unless you take the time to ask those around you how they perceive you, you can only guess some of the answers to their questions. If you do ask these people, write about their responses and what you thought they might say versus what they actually said.

- How do you imagine you are perceived by the following people?
    - Your Parents.
    - Each Sibling.
    - Grandparents.
    - Spouse or romantic partners.
    - Each child.
    - Coworkers you work most regularly with.
- Do you believe how they perceive you matches up with how you want them to see you?
    - I want _____ to perceive me as _____.
    - Why do you want them to perceive you this way?

How you see the world inspires the choices you make. Continue to journal the above questions and build on them. Keep noticing how you think about yourself and those around you.

Challenge negative beliefs. Make room in your thoughts for new possibilities. Observe judgments of self and others. This provides an opportunity for you to be in your life in different ways. Remember that thoughts are energy and felt in your body.

Dark Nights of the Solar Plexus

Most of the worries that wake us all up in the middle of the night are about relationships and resources. When you don't have what you need to stay safe, you naturally get scared. When you worry about loved ones, you set off alarm bells in your nervous system. It's one thing to have these uncertainties in the middle of the day since you can notice and redirect the fears or do something about them. It's quite another when they wake you up from a sound sleep.

The field of sleep psychology and neurobiology has done much research about the type of thinking patterns that leave most of humanity sitting in the dark, hugging their pillows. Some of the common threads of the research seem to indicate that the habit of thinking you engage in when you are awake works like white noise in bed, just waiting for its time to pounce at night. So, it's not just *what* you are thinking but *how* you are thinking when you are awake that affects your sleep quality.[57]

When you don't sleep well at night, you don't perform well during the day. Insomnia can lead to high anxiety and create a vicious cycle. Because of this, your nervous system is on high alert

---

57. Mao, Guo, and Rao, "Unraveling the Complex Interplay Between Insomnia, Anxiety, and Brain Networks."

until it has no other recourse but to shut you down into a state of dissociation. This most certainly affects your vagal tone.

Staying with what you can control is important. Changing how you think about things you have no control over is vital. How you develop good sleep hygiene is another. Some ways to help with sleepless nights and break a cycle of anxiety are:

- Move your body in healthy ways during the day.
- Write everything you need to do the next day on a sticky note, then put it in another room before bed.
- Take warm baths at night.
- Practice breathing exercises to calm your body.
- Shut off all screens.

Even if you have serious struggles, write them down on that sticky note. You can even list some things you can do in the morning to manage them. Then put the note in another room. Managing major stressors is a lot easier with some sleep.

If you have experienced traumatic moments at night as a child, your vagus nerve and brain are programmed to keep you safe in the same ways it did back then. This means that more than likely it is scanning for danger at bedtime because it cannot discern the past from the present. Notice whether your struggles with sleep have nothing to do with ruminations or anxious thought patterns. Listen to your body and see if these sleepless patterns have occurred over a lifetime. A trauma therapist can help sort this out with you. Identifying the struggle is the first step to healing the pain.

EXERCISE
Cooling the Solar Plexus

This exercise can be done anywhere you are at the moment: on a subway, at home, at a park, or at a coffee shop. Even if you are listening to this book as you move or are later in a meeting with an ornery boss. Solar plexus energy can be a difficult energy to soothe given its alignment with the epigastric region near the liver, pancreas, and spleen; these organs and branches of the vagus nerve can pack a punch. When on overdrive, the solar plexus chakra fires so intensely it can even affect the generally ennobled heart chakra.

Midway between the belly button and the solar plexus is a pressure point. In Chinese medicine this is call the Conception Vessel 12. It's located about five inches above your navel.

- Gently explore this area.
- You may need to feel around for a while, but you will experience it.
- Gently rest the first three fingers on this area.
- Breathe down into this region as you apply pressure.
- Breathe directly into the chakra as well.
- Be curious and just notice. Breathe.

Mind energy is body energy. As you are learning, how you think shows up heavily in your body. Notice how you think; challenge if you lean into any beliefs that you are a victim of circumstances. What you think of your world is how you are in your world. This formed identity manifests in your lifestyle and relationships. Reflecting on your beliefs of self leaves room for healing. This is grace and love.

EXERCISE
Earthing the Solar Plexus

Remember when you were a kid and laid stomach-down on the beach? If you have a chance to do that again, go for it. Back then we didn't care if our bathing suit got sandy. Maybe we can not care again. Lying on the grass can be just as grounding. As you lie prone on the earth's surface, pull a deep breath into the solar plexus and hold.

Press your forearms to the ground and lift your shoulders and chin up. Keep your belly on the ground. As a yoga asana, this would be "cobra." Stretching this very active chakra, especially as you are connected to the earth, might be exactly what your body needs.

EXERCISE
Fir Tree Massage

Staying with this chapter's theme of grounding to the earth, I want to end with an exercise that helps regulate all three chakras and the subdiaphragmatic branches of the vagus nerve. This requires your judgment as to how firmly or softly you touch your belly. Be intuitive and listen to your body.

Massaging the subdiaphragmatic portions of your system can unlock stuck energies and help things start moving again—sometimes literally. This area of your body takes many emotional, psychological, and even a few physical hits over time. As the sympathetic and dorsal branches of your body are regularly signaling your digestive system, they could use some tender, loving touch.

I call this exercise the Fir Tree Massage. If you have ever walked in the woods, you may have noticed that one of the most compelling features is the fir tree. The aroma grounds you in the space of the forest. If you rub the needles of the fir tree, you know that the texture is unforgettable This exercise is intended as another way to ground.

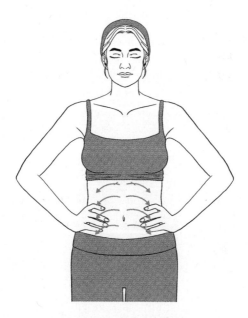

Figure 7: Fir Tree Massage

- Start by lying on your back on a place where you are comfortable.
- Rest the palms of your hands on your stomach. You can do this along the chakras or any other area that needs safe touch. This introduces a connection to your body.

- When you are ready, position fingers in a way that looks like you are getting ready to comb from the middle outward.
- Let's start at the solar plexus first.
- Rest index fingers on solar plexus with fingers in "combing" position.
- Find a firm but gentle pressure with your fingertips.
- Run your fingers outward to the edges of the rib cage.
- Then lower your combing fingers down a few inches.
- Comb from middle outward again.
- Continue "combing" your way down until you reach the root chakra.
- What do you notice?
- Afterward, you can even use your fingertips to gently roll along the edge of your rib cage.
- Work intuitively and notice how your body feels.

Summary

The chakras are reflective of the dimensions of your psychological and neurobiological reality. The chakras of the lower part of your body indicate how supported you were in childhood. They make up the root, sacral, and solar plexus energies. For this book's purpose, these chakras are called your essential dimensions because they comprise the essential parts of your human experience—from the physical to the emotional. The essential chakras connect with the subdiaphragmatic, slower-communicating fibers of the vagus nerve. These are the sympathetic and dorsal vagal branches of the vagus, which employ rest and movement. When the body experiences calm, these branches aid proper digestion of food.

When the body perceives threat, these fibers can activate a flight-or-fight response or even temporarily shut down your body.

The essential chakras, just like your vagus nerve and connecting organs, hold within them your early childhood experiences. These affect the patterns of how you connect with yourself and others now. Old experiences form your current reality. Listening to their messages through the energy they express is a wonderful way to begin healing old wounds.

Connecting to the earth, movement, and rest can be beneficial to calming your body. Growing research indicates the earth's electromagnetic field naturally quiets and balances the body's own energy field.

CHAPTER 4
YOUR HEAVENLY JOURNEY

———•———

You're now reaching the realm of human spirituality as you attune to the dimensions of what I call the evolving chakras. Evolution starts with befriending your inner experiences. It's where the collective consciousness meets individuation.[58] Here you can either develop grounded maturity or wander aimlessly in the dark, following any cluster of stars that comes along.

The ancients guided themselves by the stars, sun, and moon. They used the heavens to determine how and when to plant crops, what to forage, and how to gauge the movement of animals to hunt. Human survival was spiritually integrated into the flux of the planets. Seasonal rhythms were spiritual rhythms. Duality didn't exist. Attunement to your bodily rhythm is attunement to your divine. Opening to the luminous requires strong grounding to the essentials of your body while stretching into the essence of your divinity.

The Evolving Chakras

I call the heart, throat, third eye, and crown chakras the evolving chakras. These chakras are the entre into your subjective world, your mystical realms.

---

58. Samuels, Shorter, and Plaut, "Individuation."

The safety branch of your vagus nerve starts with the heart chakra—so does compassion, safe connection, your spiritual experiences, and empathy. The chakra energy of the heart, throat, third eye, and crown is the energy of the ventral vagal complex.

Ventral vagal (safety) nerve fibers communicate faster than the subdiaphragmatic fibers of the sympathetic (mobility) and dorsal (immobility) complexes. This is because the ventral vagal complex is myelinated, which we discussed has a fatty coating, or sheath. This safety branch modulates vocal tones, speech, and facial expressions and influences eye movement. It is what Porges calls your braking system.[59] The safety branch slows down breathing and heart rate, which lowers blood pressure and takes the body out of a reactive state. If it wasn't for this branch, your system's sympathetic nerves would keep you on overdrive.

When you feel safe, you are calm enough to engage with others. You are also able to reach deep within yourself. Breathing, stretching, humming, and engaging in bilateral movements are all ways to do this. Your heart and heart chakra make up the control center of your human management system. When you are calm, you can access all that is noble within you.

Compassion: The Heart Chakra

All roads to a compassionate existence start with the heart chakra and knowing how to access its energy. The heart chakra is at the core of love and kindness, not just for others but for yourself. Hope resides here—power too. Using heart energy to calm is always within your power now because you are learning your nervous system. Heart energy not only increases social and personal

---

59. Porges, *Polyvagal Safety*, 94.

well-being but global relief too.[60] When you work from compassion and safety, you send it outward. The heart chakra is the access point for safe social engagement through your ventral vagal complex. From a polyvagal perspective, compassion is not just about being able to soothe your own nervous system but being safely present to others—to want to act on that compassion, to help in some way, to alleviate suffering.

When you lead with compassion, you are working from a position of Soulful strength. It's no mistake that breathing is at the core of ancient spiritual practices. Now that you are aware that the breath shifts your vagal state—by increasing heart rate variably and slowing your heart rate—you can tap the brake of your "vagal car" and go the speed limit. When your body feels calm, your inner light is right there. Your breath truly is the elixir to peace. It is the opportunity to make changes for yourself and others.

EXERCISE
Hand to Heart

This is a simple exercise that helps settle your body as you circulate calm presence throughout your system. Calm might mean you need to bring your vagal state up to a more present connection with your body or settle down a more stimulated state.

- Rest your dominant hand on your heart chakra.
- Rest your nondominant hand on your root chakra.
- Pull your breath down into your root chakra and hold.
- Slowly, slowly exhale.
- Notice any shifts.

---

60. "Energetic Communication."

- Now pull your breath into your heart chakra and hold.
- Slowly, slowly exhale.
- What do you notice?

Spiritual Maturity = Vagal Intelligence

Dissociating is not calm presence. It is a patterned response from your dorsal vagal complex that perceives you are under threat. Many people who carry unresolved (and unrecognized) trauma in their body and habitually dissociate tend to perceive they are calm under pressure. There is no calm in dissociating because you are not fully present in your body. There is only disconnection from the faculties you need in that moment.

If you struggle with this, then normal stressful situations as an adult can easily activate your dorsal vagal complex. Your cognitive abilities get impaired; you have limited mobility and can't tune into your senses.[61] Emotionally you are shut off because you can't read the social cues of others. You might be slogging through the routine of your job, but you are not calm. You are simply not present.

Calm is the ability to hold safety in your body even during stressful moments. Your vagal states are both sympathetic and ventral in nature. You have enough presence through your safety state to listen, feel your body, and communicate well even under pressure.

Emotional maturity is having the capacity to be present to various feelings at once. Holding love in your body may also mean experiencing sadness or anger. Emotional maturity is the ability to allow these contradictory energies to be felt. If strong emotions were equated with childhood pain, your vagal state might

---

61. Ogden, Minton, and Pain, *Trauma and the Body*, 26.

shut down because it misreads a complex emotional experience in adulthood. Being present to a loved one's experience or expressing your own self in a safe, authentic way is an ebb and flow of vagal response and affect tolerance.

It is not unusual for people who easily dissociate—or associate physical presence with discomfort—to seek escape through the spiritual energies of the evolving chakras. Spiritual pursuits can be used to avoid problems in everyday life that need tending to. When spirituality is used to avoid emotional difficulties or the deeper work of clearing trauma, it is being used in an addictive matter called bypassing.

Imagination and creativity bring nothing but joy since they are the energy of your inner light. However, if that is the only peace you now have, reconstructing a safer physical environment outside of you might be necessary. Developing a healthy resiliency that includes a multitude of approaches is how to live in balance. In the same way emotional intelligence possesses the ability to manage several affective factors at once, spiritual maturity requires you to engage with and establish safe physical presence. Accessing the energy of your Soul energy is very much about accessing the ventral vagal complex.

Our human experiences cannot always circumvent the unexpected. As my client Tish learned, everyone, even the most spiritual seekers, must master riding the wave of the unexpected.

Tish's Story: Soul Through the Hard Parts

Tish was a local energy healer and spiritual teacher and utilized voodoo, which was part of her ancestral spiritual practices from Louisiana. She reported feeling more despondent than ever after a recent breakup with a girlfriend. At twenty-seven, Tish said she felt she was getting too old and would never find a life partner. She also said she struggled with being sexually vulnerable and had to get really high to have sex, which she believed was the cause of the breakup.

"You know," she said, "I guess I just don't like people." Her way of dealing with her fears was to shut down from everyone. If they attempted any closeness, she got aggressive. "I've got about three months of normal in me before I start getting whacky in my relationships."

"That's about the time we shift into different ways of being intimate," I said. "Less dopamine high, more emotional connection."

As she began to trust me more, Tish admitted she's felt suicidal most of her life. "Not that I'm gonna do anything about it," she said. "It just really fucks with my head."

Her way of managing when she got suicidal was to astral travel or take ayahuasca.

"I feel most at peace when I am traveling the universe during trance," she said. "People can't fuck with you then."

Tish shared that she was adopted at eighteen months old by a single white woman. "My bio mother died when I was a year old and social services was not able to find any extended family. "

I nodded.

"Mom's been a good mother." Tish shrugged. "She was able to work from home—she's in IT—so she's mostly been around while I was growing up. I have no complaints."

"Would you say you were close?"

"She struggles a lot with my spiritual practices." Tish shrugged again. "I told her in my teens I just couldn't go for that WASPy Episcopal life—no matter how liberal they claimed to be. There just wasn't anyone in Mom's world, including her, that looks like me." Tish looked up at me with a worried look that she might have offended me.

"None taken, at all." I smiled. "Growing up must have been lonely."

"Yeah, maybe," Tish said. "More like"—she paused—"untethered. I mean, I got all my needs met. My mom and me went on lots of vacations, and she provided a great education with amazing experiences. But something was missing. I felt this strongly when I got to college. That's when I eventually reached back to my cultural roots and found voodoo. It's a very comforting practice for me. Mom's not thrilled, but it's my life, not hers."

Tish struggled to be present in her day-to-day life. Despite her amazing abilities to manipulate energies, she was clearly using her spiritual practices to bypass human connection. I had to get Tish to learn about and trust her nervous system. Hers registered a lack of safety with most people she got close to. Because she struggled to be present to her affect, I wanted to start slow. We agreed to do some sessions with her mom since she was the one safe person in her life.

As Mom and daughter settled into their chairs, Tish started with a bomb of a question that I didn't see coming.

"What do you know about my birth family that I don't?" Tish looked rather smug at her mother's shock.

Mom froze. She looked to me, then Tish.

"Is this really where you want to start?" I asked Tish.

"Is there something you're afraid to tell me?" Tish crossed her arms and looked at her mother.

A long pause filled the room.

"I can't," her mother said. "It would be too horrible for you to know." Her mother went pale and looked to me for help.

"Tish?" I said. "Your mom is clearly trying to protect you from something. Do you really want to know what it is?"

"Whatever it is, I feel it anyway." She looked at me. "From all the somatic work we've been doing, I know that information is stored in my body." She turned back to her mother. "What is it, Mom?"

Slowly and through tears, Tish's mother revealed Tish had been molested by her father after her mother died. "He was your only surviving family and social services took you away."

"Well." Tish looked at me with guarded sarcasm. "Like I hadn't figured something like that was coming."

"The first time I saw you, I wanted you," Tish's mother said. "You were so sweet and sassy. But a little withdrawn. It was like even back then you were challenging me to love you."

Tish's shoulders softened.

"I truly want that challenge, Tish." Her mom's eyes filled with tears. "I hope I haven't been a disappointment."

The sarcastic edge softened in Tish's large eyes. She glanced to me, then turned back to her mother. "Thanks for that," she whispered. "Seriously, Mom, thanks."

The next session Tish came by herself. "I'm ready," she said. "I think I can do this."

Tish's first task was to trust her body in movement. We took plenty of walks around the lake and worked to engage her sympathetic vagal branch in fun ways. I introduced her to Brainspotting and Internal Family Systems work. The more she was able to connect with and help unburden the many inner children who worked hard to protect her all these years, the calmer she was becoming.

Over time, Tish began to feel safe enough in her body to process that implicit memory. On her own, Tish started yoga. Her demeanor from our first session to nine months later had changed.

She was calm, still her hysterically sarcastic self, but in a happier and less defensive way. I have seen Tish off and on for years now. Her mystic arts and astral traveling are being done in different ways.

"I'm not trying to get the hell out of here anymore," she said. "I'm not lying around high, trying to convince myself I am seeking the answers to the universe." She rested a hand on her chest. "The answers are in here. I actually like being in my body now."

Connection: The Throat Chakra

Words matter. They are a vibrational frequency with intention. They can heal and connect, or they can harm and create pain. Along with how we speak, how we listen is tied to the energy around the throat chakra. Polyvagal theory discusses how the middle ear fibers can shift depending on the need to listen for safety cues.[62] Tone of voice also matters, as your system is designed to respond in safety to a midrange of tone that is called prosody in polyvagal theory. High tones or very low voice frequencies put our systems in defensive modes.

The throat chakra is one of the more complex and interesting of the chakra energy centers. The energy runs along and into the throat and up to the ears. The flow then cycles back around. When we think of the throat chakra, we think of speaking. But without the ability to listen, sound makes very little difference.

The throat possesses the bilateral fibers that run on both the left and the right sides of the larynx and pharynx. This region of ventral vagal nerve endings is helping you interact with others through the jaw, tongue, and middle ear.

---

62. Porges, *Polyvagal Safety*, 74.

The throat chakra is the only energy center that can be used with full intention. It is the energy of relatedness and expresses itself through various tones and frequencies. It is also abused with false speech and hurtful sound.

With this ability to manifest vibration and language, Soul can express itself in ways that the other energy centers cannot.

Song and musical resonances are some of the ways. The painful wailing of the banshee is the imprint of loss on the Soul. In the Buddhist eight-fold path, right speech encourages no lying, idle chatter, rude words, or telling one person what another has said about them.[63]

EXERCISE
Hum Like a Child Again

Yep, it can be that easy. Humming gets you into your natural range of prosody and calms your body. Just like breathing, humming engages the ventral vagal safety fibers of the vagus nerve.

Before, during, and after you hum, notice your body and its state. Then hum for as long and as loud as you want to.

- What is your favorite song?
- Go ahead and hum it.
- Do you like to make up tunes?
- Go for it.

---

63. Bodhi, *The Noble Eightfold Path*, 12.

Mystery of Your Soul Through Sound

Your Soul has a natural tug toward a higher principle, and when you are humming, you can feel it. Listen and allow the vibration to course your body. It will lead you. When you listen inside, you are hearing your internal music. When you listen outside, certain words or tones and even music complement that resonance.

The pull toward your guiding principles starts getting a little cacophonous when you repeat old, destructive behaviors or when you cannot identify what your needs are. When fears that are not actually present override you, it's difficult to experience your natural vibration. You're wandering in a noisy room and can't hear your own voice. Suddenly, that simple Soulful compass starts feeling like a complicated GPS system with directions spoken in another language.

When this happens, step back and let the simplicity of your vibration recalibrate. Press your hand to your heart. Breathe deep and hum. Tap into what you need. Take your time. That's how you manage your inner world. Slowly attune to your body, and honor the Soul's rhythm.

Spirituality: The Third Eye Chakra

The third eye chakra sits between your brows and just above it. This chakra is the visionary eye that rests between your three-dimensional seeing eyes. It flows to and from your prefrontal cortex. The prefrontal cortex is the higher reasoning portion of your brain. It brings in big concepts, wider perspectives, and engages you with your imaginal world.

Just as the ventral vagal branch of the vagus nerve feels like the key that opens you to the warmth of your Soul, the prefrontal cortex and third eye chakra are a canvas for the Soul. The Soul is kind and intuitive. It wants to say something to humankind in better ways. The Soul's language is symbolic. It speaks using motifs, ideas, and impressions. The third eye is its outlet.

Ocular nerve fibers intricately connect your eyes to your brain and the vagus nerve. I have mentioned bilateral stimulation. This is a back-and-forth movement of the eyes. Bilateral movement is what your eyes do in REM (rapid eye movement) sleep. This is when we dream. The REM stage of sleep is vital for us to process the events of our life and reconsolidate memories in our system. This processing fully engages the energy of the third eyes as well, since the dream experience is not a literal one but a visionary one.

Opening and using the energy of the third eye can take work when we are not sleeping. Since our awake mind naturally engages in scanning for dangers, it can easily stimulate warning signs to the sympathetic branches of the vagus and active the solar plexus. Be patient with yourself and breathe into this tension.

EXERCISE
Bilateral Tapping

Bilateral tapping is like a gentle rolling of your insides. It engages the left, then right hemisphere of both your brain and your vagus nerve. When this happens, all organs feel this calm.

Slow, gentle taps are what we want here. Not fast taps. I would highly discourage fast taps since they will generally stimulate your system, not calm it. Fast is what we do when trauma therapists are in the midst of helping a client work through their traumatic event using Eye Movement Desensitization Reprocessing (EMDR). Slow taps provide what feels like a calm, loving rocking effect. It's very easy and you might be naturally doing this anyway. Here is how to break this down.

- Just rest a hand on each thigh.
- Start by slowly and gently tapping the top of one leg, then the other leg.
- Bring your breath down into your lungs and release gradually on the exhale.
- Just sit and tap. One leg and then the other leg.

Growth and Change

When you grow, everything around you changes. That's because you are different. When you begin to know yourself, you begin to individuate.[64] This means you start to know who you are outside of your family, cultural background, and even friends. As a result, you may find your new authenticity is disturbing to some people who are used to your old ways. As you settle deeper into your own way of being, you will eliminate old beliefs, old ways of communicating, old friends, and old patterns. Trust this growth by deepening into who you already are.

Knowing ourselves is the one thing we all want, yet it's the one thing we all fear. Change starts with trusting your inner world. When you change on the inside, you eventually change on the outside. The outside seems to be where we get stuck. It's lonely when the people around us no longer see things the same way we do. However, it also goes against the grain of our Souls not to evolve.

Individuation has been distrusted by organizations for centuries. This shows itself today in places where people who do not believe the same way are subjugated. Part of inward work is allowing yourself to feel in ways you may have been avoiding because they were inconvenient for you or the people around you.

---

64. Samuels, Shorter, and Plaut, "Individuation."

The only way to find the truth of your spirit is to stop listening to how others want to shape you and begin to let your Soul take the lead. There is one universal, absolute truth, and that is that the truth lies within each and every one of us. That truth is both the same and different for all of us, and that is okay.

Empathy: The Crown Chakra

At its core, empathy is a vibration. It is a finer, fuller frequency that—just like every other frequency on this planet—is felt. Vibrational patterns are produced from one human being to another. Empathy is one of the most noble of these energies.

While the connection that creates empathy is a heart-generated one, that experience expands to the mind and into the crown chakra as meaning is made. When the mind responds (in calmness) to the loving-kindness of the empathetic frequency, that energy is sent outward into the universal web of connection.[65]

The crown chakra energy rests between the prefrontal lobe and the parietal lobe of your brain and the front and parietal bones of the skull. It is where your soft spot, the fontanel, was as an infant. It has been discussed in Buddhist traditions that this is the portal by which the Soul enters and leaves the body. According to Paramahansa Yogananda in his classic book *Autobiography of a Yogi* and other Buddhist masters, the fontanel softens again as we die and at times of death displays a cerebrospinal fluid.[66] Cerebrospinal fluid is a clear fluid that cushions the brain and spinal cord. It carries nutrients and regulates the pressure in the brain. It even helps protect the brain from infection. It replenishes and cleanses,

---

65. "Energetic Communication."
66. Yogananda, *Autobiography of a Yogi*; Sogyal, *The Tibetan Book of Living and Dying*.

carrying toxins from the nervous system. The cerebrospinal fluid responds to light, vibration, hormones, ions, and molecules.[67] It is in constant flux, and its health is influenced by many factors, including diet.

We are made of more than 90 percent water when we are born. When we die, that percentage drops close to 50 percent. According to the research of Masura Emoto, the message of water is love and gratitude.[68] Water flows through us as a vehicle of communication.

Consider that your crown chakra may be the master at pulling spiritual messages into your system from above The core of spiritual "downloads" are full of love, as they are from a plane of existence you might have disconnected from during your human travails. Because all your energy centers both generate and receive information, opening your crown chakra opens your whole system up to the beneficent frequencies of the universe.

Holding Space

Felt experience, not thought, is what expands and matures us. Presence to others is the access point to developing an ability to connect and show you care about them. Empathy is not taking on another's energy. That is just bad boundaries. We are not stronger together when we allow someone's discharged pain to infiltrate our own system. Rescuing is not empathy. Rescuing is a form of control with the intention that the rescuer feel some power.

Holding space in your body is feeling safe enough within your own system to be present to another's pain. This is one of the highest human experiences. Remaining present and connected

---

67. Zappaterra, "Connection to Source via the Cerebrospinal Fluid."
68. Emoto, *The Hidden Messages in Water*, 134.

is the ability to breathe and stay connected to your ventral vagal complex. This creates enough space between us and others so they can be seen and heard and we can listen.

Magnetoreception

We have extensive language that describes our physical place in the world and the ways our body gauges it. *Interoception* is the neurobiological term for sensing your internal response to external stimuli. Exteroception is the external biological perception of your body's placement in the world. *Neuroception*, a term coined by Porges, is the nervous system's response to stimuli before we have an awareness of it.

So, let's talk about *magnetoreception*. This sense helps creatures detect the earth's magnetic field. It's an experience that allows living beings to orient and navigate. You can see this each season with birds that migrate. They possess a cranial nerve in their beaks that helps them navigate back to the same places. Many marine animals, including sharks and turtles, do too. This nerve, which is composed of the mineral iron, seems to attune to the magnetic frequencies of the planet. Radio frequencies can scramble this communication. There have been enough news stories over the years, with flocks of birds, pods of whales and other species showing up in places they would not inhabit before. Scientists have surmised it was because these frequencies got scrambled.

Given that humans are also creatures that inhabit this earth, does it not make sense we, too, have magnetic draws to places? That we experience magnetoreception? Scientists are still wondering whether different species possess different sensors depending on a draw to the south or north pole or even the equator. The scientific community posits that there is still much discussion as to whether humans can sense the magnetic frequencies of the earth, though we do have our own facial structures that respond to the frequencies. Our retinas and the ethmoid bone, found in the nose, possess magnetic material. Our alpha brainwaves are also affected.[69]

Given that our neurobiology and chakras emit an electromagnetic frequency that has been measured by some scientists, why wouldn't we feel certain pulls toward places, people, and experiences of home?[70] Certainly, our logical mind and reductionist tendencies try to override these natural impulses, though I wonder if those efforts ever really block out that magnetoreception. I believe we are drawn to others' frequencies, to communities, and places we might have never been to before but intuitively know. Each chakra plays a role in this because each plexus of nerves stores memories as the Soul generates the call.

EXERCISE
Opening to the Lotus

Get comfortable and sit in a position where you can focus on the energies at the top of your skull. If you need to, rest a palm on your head to connect to this energy. I personally find this helps to charge my crown chakra. As you sit, imagine a comforting shawl around your shoulders. Let its color be a calm and safe hue for you. This shawl can be as long or as short as you need it to be. The objective is to have you feel a soft enfolding around you. This is a form of earthly protection as you reach outward.

---

69. Wang et al., "Transduction of the Geomagnetic Field as Evidenced from Alpha-Band Activity in the Human Brain."
70. Chae et al., "Human Magnetic Sense Is Mediated by a Light and Magnetic Field Resonance-Dependent Mechanism."

Breathe through your nostrils. Pull the air into the midsection of your skull. If you struggle with this, soften your jaw, as this will relieve tension in the skull muscles.

- Repeat the following statement in your mind: "I open to the energies of universal benevolence."
- Sit for a while as you connect and perceive the energy around you.
- Be the curious observer of this experience.
- What are the physical sensations? Are you receiving information? Are you experiencing colors or energies?
- Do you see guides, angels, or other benevolent beings? If so, what are they sharing?
- When you are done, thank any guides, images, or symbols you see.
- As you finish up this exercise, don't just get up and move, as you may need to ground. Wiggle your goes, move your feet in circles, engage your hips with soft rolling movement. This calls in your leg muscles as a reminder to be present. Make sure you always ground in your body before you get up and move.

EXERCISE
Heart to Crown Synergy

If you have been doing many of the exercises in this chapter, you will be in a good place to work through this next one. This engages ventral vagal safety branches of your nervous system with the synergistic flow of the crown chakra. I think I can confidently say that you will experience a profound shift in your energy after this exercise, especially if you keep doing this on a daily basis.

- Sit comfortably.
- Pull in deep breaths, as we have practiced in previous chapters.
- Slowly exhale through your mouth (remember the flute breath).
- At the same time as the exhale, keep your jaw muscles soft. This creates more access to throat, face, and skull energy as it sends signals of safety.
- Continue this breathing pattern. Notice if you feel a sense of calm and safety in your body.
- Your heart rate will slow, even as you feel more exhilarated.
- Pull deep breaths and fill your lungs. This automatically expands heart chakra energy.
- Once you feel attuned to your heart chakra and ventral vagal branch, keep breathing like this and shift attention to your crown chakra.
- Slowly continue to do your "flute" breathing as you connect more deeply with the crown chakra energy. Take your time.
- Stay here for as long as you need to.
- Just notice any shifts in your body.

You can make this a regular practice. It can be as formal or casual as you like. This can be applied as you meditate or just sit in a chair. If this helps you alleviate anxiety, then by all means continue this. If this alleviates tension, then that is fantastic. The outcome is unique to you. There is no right or wrong.

Summary

The evolving chakras are the beginning of the ventral vagal complex of your vagus nerve. This branch aligns with your heart, lungs, throat, and middle ears. It acts as a brake that can slow down and modulate the rest of your system. These nerve fibers affect how well you connect to your present moment experiences, and they increase your ability to be present to others in times of stress. This is the nerve complex that generates a sense of safety in your body. It's safety that brings you to spirituality, which allows you to access your Soul energy.

The chakra dimensions of the heart (compassion), throat (connection), third eye (spirituality), and crown (empathy) align along this region of your body. While the third eye and crown chakras connect more to cranial fibers and align with ventricles—or spaces—that hold cerebral spinal fluid in your brain, they also send signals to the vagal complex through other nerve pathways.

Ventral vagal fibers of safety are faster moving than the subdiaphragmatic fibers of the sympathetic (mobility) and dorsal (immobility) branches. These safety fibers rapidly send signals throughout your system. This quick communication is what can immediately slow things down so you can regain balance.

PART 2
THE WAY FORWARD

CHAPTER 5
PAYING ATTENTION WHILE DRIVING

$\bullet\!\!-\!\!\!-\!\!\!-\!\!\bullet$

When I write, I envision the readers I am writing for. I imagine people who are seeking, trying various ways to manage their lives, and attempting to learn from each new experience they have. I see them as psychologically and spiritually curious, happy, struggling, sad, confused, mourning, doubting, or excited. Maybe they're a ways down the path on their trauma healing, or maybe they are just beginning. I imagine that all of you reading this right now are learning to be okay with not always being okay (always a toughie).

I also see people who struggle with escapism from the difficulties in their lives. Life is full of what we call trauma. Losing a pet can impact your world as strongly as losing a job. Neglect in childhood impacts you as much as enmeshed parents who can't honor your privacy. Loneliness and fear are hard to endure but are too many times part of the human condition we must sit with.

Whomever I believe I am writing to, I desire to share the fact that being human is sometimes hard. Even when you've "got this" and especially if you came into life with instability from caretakers, you will hit potholes. You are not alone. We are all weary travelers. Even the people who look like they are rolling along just fine have struggles we can't see. We all have to keep our eyes on the road while we drive this journey of life.

Paying attention at the wheel means not swerving around the tender spots. Avoiding old pain, rather than accepting it's there, is bypassing.[71] Admitting you carry woundedness in your body is the start to healing. It's also surprisingly hard to do, especially when you have spent a lifetime building a persona of authority around those wounds. How do you even open to the idea that you have unhealed pain if it has been squashed down? How do you balance a spiritual practice with a psychological healing path? Did choosing a healing profession make you assume you could heal others as a way to heal yourself? It didn't for me. I still had my own work to do and continue to do so, by the way.

People who bypass are looking for a fast fix. They come into my office but don't stay long if they are not open to the sometimes slow process of attuning to their body as a source of guidance. It's not possible to heal—trauma or otherwise—and be dissociated from your human experience.

Not that learning to be present should be a brutally harsh experience that forces you to relive traumatic memories. That is exactly the opposite work a trained trauma therapist does. We are aware that many people fear being present transports them back to their pain. Healing trauma is just like being present to and process-ing your grief (which can be a form of trauma). You lean in; you lean out.[72] In trauma processing, we take our time and understand that resolving the old pains we carry is an unfolding. It's not a neat, mental, linear process with a perfect beginning, middle, and end. Boy, how I wish that was the case. I would gladly work my way out of a job. Every day.

---

71. Welwood, *Toward a Psychology of Awakening*.
72. Pearlman et al., *Treating Traumatic Bereavement*, 121.

A lifetime of dents and bruises didn't happen overnight. The journey to reparation needs to have a pace that is unique to your own pattern of healing. If you haven't taken on noticing and healing your trauma, how could you even understand what your pace looks like? Holding space for yourself by avoiding polarities, such as right versus wrong, means walking a middle way. Buddhists call this the way of the dharma, or teachings of the Buddha.

Taking the middle way means not taking sides with yourself. Not being good. Not being bad. Just be curious. Being the curious observer of your neurobiology means willing to be impartial. Taking out the "why" parks that old narrative that's been driving you for so long. When you do this, you can learn to be compassionate with yourself. When "why" no longer keeps defenses up—as in "why did this happen?" or "why did they hurt me?"—then "how" can sit beside you. In other words, asking "how" brings in a way forward. It empowers you. Then questions you ask about your healing are different:

- How does my body feel?
- How am I experiencing this moment?
- How am I wanting to respond?
- How am I observing what is occurring?
- How can I heal these wounds?

"How" brings you to presence. You are in the moment in a way that provides personal power. Being in the moment keeps you inquisitive. This is where your healing starts. This is the practice of mindfulness.[73]

---

73. Goldstein, *Mindfulness*, 256.

What Is Mindfulness?

Mindfulness is a practice of awareness that comes from the Buddhist traditions. It is not a religious practice. It is a psychological one that brings you spiritual peace.

Buddhist traditions span a good two thousand years or more. Like any other belief, Buddhism has branched off into various practices across the globe. The term *mindfulness*, or *sati*,[74] stems from the Pali tradition of Buddhism. Pali is the ancient language of the Theravada school of Buddhism. It is an Indo-Aryan Language. *Sati* means to be aware, to cultivate present moment attention to thoughts, sensations, and emotions without judgment.

Thanks to many Western psychologists and other mental health practitioners who spent decades practicing Buddhist disciplines, therapeutic approaches now have a strong foundation of mindfulness. Jon Kabat-Zinn was instrumental in developing Mindfulness-Based Stress Reduction (MBSR). Mindfulness-Based Relapse Prevention (MBRP) is used in treatment centers and came from Washington state. Two cognitive-based mindfulness approaches are Mindfulness-Based Cognitive Therapy (MBCT) and Acceptance Commitment Therapy (ACT). These approaches have helped people manage depression, anxiety, eating disorders, and personality disorders.[75] They have given a foundation for people to approach life from a kinder, more curious way that allows for self-awareness and self-patience.

The mindfulness approach took a secular turn in the 1980s and 90s. Ideological and religious beliefs of Buddhism were set aside to the make the practice of awareness more psychological in its approach. Insight meditation, Vipassana, is what I use

---

74. Batchelor, *After Buddhism*, 333.
75. Linehan, *DBT Skills*.

as a framework throughout this book when I share mindfulness exercises.

Vipassana is a loving, kind interest to what is in your heart and mind.[76] Through awareness of thoughts and breath and inquiring into your personal experience, you can apply non-judgment. Being curious helps you access you. A safe and compassionate approach to self and others is at the heart of insight meditation. This is also the way to gauge your neuroception. Kindly observing takes the shame out of it. There is a right and true power in observing one-self. Let's start with some very simple but powerful exercises to get you used to integrating mindfulness into your everyday life.

EXERCISE
Mindful Walking

Mindful walking is an attunement to how you are feeling inter-nally as well as how you experience the outside world. It's not about the end goal. The power comes from being present on the journey. Don't rush when you walk. This is about being in the moment.

I live in an older part of my town, and the sidewalks some-times feel like forest pathways given how the concrete has worn over time. I have to notice the next step while paying attention to how my feet are feeling on the uneven pavement. I found this to be a good way to sum up being present as you walk. It's observing. It's awareness without fear.

- As you step outside, take a moment.
- Draw in a deep breath.
- Connect to the sights and sounds.

---

76. Goldstein and Kornfield, *Seeking the Heart of Wisdom*, 7.

- Breathe air into your body.
- Stand straight to let the energy flow along your spine.
- Look around you.
- Are you in a familiar environment?
- Look at an everyday detail that you might not have seen before.
- Does your neighbor's roof line slope in a way you have never noticed? What does the bark look like on that tree you pass by every day?
- Slowly stretch your arms and legs.
- Notice any tightness.
- Give yourself time to feel the blood rushing to the areas as you stretch.
- How does the energy feel?
- Notice the sky.
- Attune to the sounds around you. Are they seasonal? Does your winter sound different from how your spring sounds?
- Slowly take another breath.
- How does the air feel against your skin?
- As you walk, listen.
- Are there cars?
- How do the trees sound? Listen for birds.
- How are your feet feeling as you step?
- How do your shoulders and arms feel?
- Notice the temperature of the air. Is it cool or warm?
- How does the air feel on your face? How does it feel going into your nostrils, throat, and lungs?
- How are you noticing your energy as you do this everyday movement?

Your Vagus Nerve in Real Time

As you walk, you incorporate the most built-in bilateral experience you have: one leg, then the other. You use your arms in a natural sway. Your movement balances out the sacrum, the spine, and the skull. As your hips align, the other parts of your system naturally respond. When your skeletal system finds balance and more adaptability with movement, your nervous system adjusts too. So do your organs. Your whole internal communication network engages in the ways it was designed to.

Walking balances out more than body alignment. It releases endorphins. Your heart rate increases, and your lung capacity grows, which strengthens ventral vagal (safety branch) health as you engage sympathetic (mobility) branches.

Because you are walking at a calm pace and being intentional about the sensations in and around you, your system releases a balance of hormones. If you struggle with adrenal fatigue, regular mindful walking is one of the best ways to restore your whole nervous system. You are moving, which your body is asking for, without overstimulating it.

Your Chakras in Real Time

As you walk, you are actively engaging with the energy of the chakras, as movement innervates all the branches of your vagus nerve. The energy that runs down your legs from the root chakra feels that flow. Your pulse increases and lung capacity is challenged, opening up the heart and throat chakras. The root, sacral, and solar plexus chakras are all engaged in the movement.

★ ★ ★

Perhaps you don't walk regularly, so the mindful walking exercise may take some time to feel comfortable. When we are sedentary or have been injured, the body alters to a more immobile state. Muscles tighten to accommodate pain, which skews the skeletal system and eventually pinches or shortens the nerves. The organs are not getting the blood and oxygen support they need. Certainly, our car-influenced society keeps us from walking the miles our ancestors did. Regaining connection to movement means walking needs to be started slowly, intentionally, and without strict rules. Enjoy.

That Healthy Tension

Being mindful of how you are interacting in your world has a tension to it. Learning to be okay with momentarily not being okay is that present moment mastery I keep talking about. Whether your tension comes from sadness, loneliness, annoyance, or guilt, just breathe. Notice your thoughts about these emotions without trying to fix them. Breathe some more.

If the affect is strong, try looking outside yourself for grounding or safety cues. As if you have just finished a steep climb up a mountain passage, stand back. Inhale. Observe where you are. Let that breathing reset your system. Notice. Accept.

Every one of us experiences struggles. It's how we manage them that leads you to a healthier, more balanced life. I have personally reminded myself, when I am hurting, that others are struggling too. This is not to minimize my own pain but to remind myself that being human has its struggles and no one is immune.

When the struggle arises, know this moment won't last forever, that this is a fleeting experience you are willing to be curious about. Whether your past is intruding into the present, your racing thoughts are making you believe things that are not real, or there is an inexplicable discomfort in your body, your breath is the entry point to working with that tension.

Let yourself be present to it.

EXERCISE
Mindful Listening

This exercise can be done while walking, and I'm encouraging you to do so. This can also be done—and has a different experience—when you are still. Listening mindfully can be done anytime.

When you are alone, slow your pace. If you are driving, slow to the speed limit and notice what you hear. If you're walking, slow and notice the sounds of your steps. Remember the neurobiological changes in your ear middle based on polyvagal theory. If you perceive you will be late and need to rush, then your body is not feeling safe. Your middle ear shifts how it listens then. If you slow down and lower your heart rate, your middle ear listens differently.

You can be doing or "non-doing," as Jon Kabat-Zinn calls it,[77] and still direct your curiosity to the sounds around you. Whether you are sitting quietly or cleaning the dishes, pay attention. Listening brings an awareness to things that might even make you see, feel, and sense differently. As you listen, notice:

- How are you experiencing your neighborhood sounds?
- What sounds are you noticing that you didn't before?
- What sounds are you hearing that are close to you?

---

77. Kabat-Zinn, *Wherever You Go, There You Are*.

- What sounds are you hearing that are off in the distance?
- Do any of these sounds surprise you?
- Are there people nearby?
- If so, what do their voices sound like?
- How are you experiencing your body as you hear these voices?

Listening upon Waking

When you first wake up, spend a few minutes listening. Your body is still in a restful state, so it is perceiving things in a way that it doesn't during the middle of your day. Perhaps you hear these sounds so frequently that you barely pay attention. Perhaps these sounds are integrated so fully into your waking routine they are signaling your system to wake up and you stop noticing them.

- What do you notice?
- How do the sheets sound as you move?
- How are you breathing?
- What does it feel like?
- Can you hear neighbors?
- Birds?
- What season are you in?
- How does winter or summer sound in your home?
- How do the seasons sound outside?
- What about fall or spring?
- Do you have a heater or air conditioner on?
- Can you hear anyone else in your home?

Three-Tiered Listening

Listening while you are alone allows you to apply what I call a three-tiered approach. Do this once with eyes open and again with them closed and notice if you have a different experience.

The First Tier—The first tier is where the more overt sounds are. Think of dogs barking, trucks rolling by, laundry machines humming, or people talking loudly. Listen in a way that makes you wonder. For example, you may hear your neighbor outside every morning. Be curious and ask yourself these questions. Also, as always, notice how your body feels as you do this.

- What are the people near you saying?
- What is the quality of their voice?
- What emotion is in their voice?
- How fast or slowly are they speaking?
- What are you feeling in your body as you listen?

The Second Tier—At the second tier are the sounds behind the sounds. Are the people talking doing something that creates its own sound, like shuffling their feet, washing dishes, or doing yard work? Do you hear trees rustling or birds chirping?

- Breathe and listen.
- What are you feeling in your body as you listen?

The Third Tier—The third tier drops you down a little deeper. As you focus on the less overt sounds, your body slows down. Sometimes these sounds are within us. Sometimes they are far away, outside of us, and we would not normally notice them. Notice how it shifts as listening to the third tier of sounds requires you to be more still.

- Breathe.
- Do you hear the air being pulled into your lungs?
- Do you hear your heartbeat?
- Does the sound of the beat match the feel of the beat?
- Do you hear ringing in your ears?
- Is your stomach softly gurgling?
- Pull attention to outside of you and listen beyond the obvious sounds.
- What do you notice?
- Is there an animal scratching in the distance?
- Are there aircraft way overhead?
- Can you hear any sounds of leaves? Or trees outside?

Listening to Others

We've been listening to ourselves as part of these exercises. Now, let's practice listening to others. The next time you are with someone, slow down and pay attention in ways you may not have before. To begin with, don't listen to answer—or notice if you are wanting to answer and how it feels in your body. Truly drop down into paying attention to what they are saying and how they are communicating. Don't respond with words, but feel free to engage with your body language to affirm you are present to them.

- What do you notice about how this person is speaking?
- How are they breathing as they speak?
- Where are they looking as they talk to you?

- What is the tone of their voice?
- Does that tone shift as they change subjects?
- What is their expression like?
- Does that expression change as they are speaking?

As you are hearing them, apply your mindfulness skills to how your own body is experiencing them.

- What do you notice about your body?
- Where are you feeling energy?
- How are you positioned as you listen?
- Is your body tense? Relaxed?
- How does the expression on your face feel?
- Are you wanting to talk?
- What does that feel like in your body?
- How safe does your body feel?

Sometimes, what we say is very different from how we say things.[78] Tone and body language matter and can be driven by your nervous system without you understanding it. Be mindful of felt experience as you increase awareness of others.

The Collective Vagal Listening Experience

When you are with people, your vagus nerve is on point. It is gauging and interpreting before you are aware of it (neuroception). Your body may respond with a twinge, jolt, eye blink, or frown before your brain and conditioned social skills can filter the reaction.

---

78. Porges and Porges, *Our Polyvagal World*, 63.

Here's the catch: The nervous systems you are with are also doing the same. Imagine this rapid, collective "reading of the room" during a party:

People are gathering. Their nervous systems are already making meaning of how safe they feel way before they can understand the messages coming from their bodies. Not everyone is going to have the same internal experience because the vagus and brain always consider past experiences for present protection. As the people enter the space, everyone is having a neurobiological conversation with themselves. As they come into contact with others, briefly, no one is speaking exactly the same language.

Over time, people identify what their stomachs, facial expressions, or muscles are doing and feeling as they make sense of this gathering and how safe they feel in it. In this case, neuroception makes way for interoception, which is awareness of how your body feels as a result of external experiences. The partygoers now begin to seek out others they like. Words are spoken, stories are shared, and gestures of warmth and acceptance are made. As people feel safe, the room begins to coalesce with a unified energy.

Through the polyvagal perspective, how you listen has neurobiological qualities.[79] In other words, listening is a felt experience. Now that you understand your nervous system rapidly flows with information, you can honor the shifting energies in ways you have never done before. You can also extend a proverbial "ear" to those who are struggling by being safe in your own body in order to help them feel regulated with you.

All this being said, your literal ears are greatly affected by the phylogenetic shifts of your nervous system. The vagus collaborates with other cranial nerves to make this happen. Your inner

---

79. Porges and Porges, *Our Polyvagal World*, 20–22.

ear is deeply connected to the central nervous system through the brain stem and contributes to balance and hearing. Your middle ear muscles, through the indirect messages of your ventral or sympathetic fibers, can act like a camera aperture, opening and closing in response to the sounds around you.

Go back to that party. Imagine everyone has found a friend or small circle of people to speak with. The cheerful humming of other voices does not affect how they listen to the people they are laughing with. That is because the ventral fibers have registered safety, and the ear muscles have narrowed to "tune in." Now imagine a large bang in the middle of the room. The people stop talking; their sympathetic branches engage to make way for a run or possible fight. Everyone's middle ear muscles have opened to accommodate the environmental sounds around them.

Your listening shifts as the environment changes around you. This includes how you hear voices. In polyvagal theory, the term *prosody* is used to describe the rhythm, tone, or pitch of a voice that conveys emotional meaning. A midrange tone in a person's voice signals an experience of safety. High-pitched ranges send signals of possible danger. Lower pitches are also an indication of lack of safety. Imagine someone you enjoy speaking in a calm voice. Now notice how this feels in your body.

Your Listening Chakras

Each chakra listens because it is an extension of your nervous system. These energies are both emitted and received, absorbed back into the system as a felt sense. When your body is safe, it eases. This is when you can more easily tune in to and "listen" to the flow of your energy centers.

Your essential chakras of root, sacral, and solar plexus are how you can hear the vibrations of nature, patterns of the weather, and rhythms of the seasons. Listening through stillness as well as movement is how we have been designed to stay connected to the places that sustain us and foster our safety.

The evolving chakras of heart, throat, third eye, and crown call out and listen for frequencies of love and Soulful guidance. How well the body is harbored by the essentials of life indicates what is said and how it is heard. These energies are aligned not only with the vagus nerve but many other cranial nerves. This means that these chakras also play an energetic front line in your basic human defense of chewing and digesting food. And there is nothing more basic than the ability to smell what is consumed before it is eaten. That sense of smell improves when the body is safe and out of threat mode. Sometimes, pulling in scent is what takes your system out of an arousal state. The following is a mindfulness exercise that can help.

EXERCISE
Mindful Smelling

This mindful smelling exercise is different from the mindful breathing exercises throughout this book. This exercise is truly about the act of smelling. The one sensory experience you cannot explain to others but has the most profound impact on your Soul is smell. Scents inspire both implicit (felt) and explicit (remembered) memories. When scents connect with memories that are happy, you can be immediately transported to a loving time and place. When scents are associated with pain and fear, that transportation is scary and can contribute to traumatic flashbacks.

New smells and pleasant old scents can build resiliency as you work your life back to safety.

For instance, do you love the scent of a freshly cut apple? How about a grilled steak? Or a pot of soup? How does your system respond when you smell a newborn baby's skin? What about the nutty scent of a kitten? Fresh bread? Pine trees? Sea air? The wind? A coffee shop?

For this next exercise, I want you to start by making a list for each prompt:

- What are the scents from childhood that made me happy?
- What are the scents from childhood that made me calm?
- What are the memories I enjoyed?
- What scents make me feel safe now?
- What scents have I been curious about?

Spend time consciously engaged in smelling. Find a store with natural oils and explore new smells. Pick a scent that calms and a scent that invigorates.

Consider the elements of a scent. For instance, you might love the scents from the element of fire. Find incenses of woods that you can burn that bring you to safety. You may be drawn to earth energy, so grasses, flowers, or salts might be what you need around you. Oils and diffusers help if you are drawn to the element of water. Fresh trees and a cool breeze might be the air element scents you desire.

As you add scents into your life that bring safety to your body, notice what changes occur in the moment and over time.

Your Vagus Nerve

Olfactory nerves derive from your first cranial nerve (remember that the vagus nerve is the tenth cranial nerve). The primary olfactory nerve intersects with a variety of cortical and limbic structures in your brain that hold memories. What this means is smells easily conjure past experiences, then those memories signal from the brain down to the vagus nerve. As you are now aware, safety is a primary concern for the vagus. One way or another, scents will affect your neuroception.

Your Chakras

Because scent inspires memories, the experience of smelling can very much be a heart chakra opening or closing. If the smell is pleasant, then the heart, throat, and even third eye energies will easily flow. If the smell brings back a scary memory, all energy intensifies because your body orients toward survival. If the memory is charged with danger and flashbacks occur, sympathetic engagement of the nervous system lights the chakras up like an overloaded electrical system. Be gentle if you get activated in these ways by scents and know it is not a character flaw that you reacted, but there is some solid science behind why you feel discomfort. This is an indication that you can provide some deep self-care for your system.

* * *

If a scent stimulates a traumatic response, take yourself out of the environment that is charging you. Call a safe person. Find a place to ground yourself. Pull out a scent that creates a calming, safe experience for you.

When I first start working with a client, I introduce them to essential oils and have them on hand during the sessions. Clients will generally know what scents feel good for them, then purchase their own. I have learned so much through the years from my clients. Some that love peppermint smells carry mints. Some that love shampoo smells or lotions will have a small bottle in their purse. Some even put air fresheners in their car that involve happy memories. Find what your "happy" smells are and keep them within reach.

EXERCISE
Mindful Eating

Eating is at the core of your survival, yet it becomes an over-charged experience if messages around food consumption reflect feelings of your lovability and worthiness.

Mindful eating is about being fully present to preparing and consuming food. In this way, you are caring for yourself by slowing things down. From the texture and the taste of the food to the experience of sitting with and eating the food, going slow brings new awareness to an everyday process.[80]

If you struggle with disordered eating or eating disorders, even pleasant smells of food will set your alarm bells off. As you mindfully prepare your food in this exercise, pay attention to the affect in your body. Notice what thoughts, feelings, or beliefs arise.

- Before you eat, prepare a place at the table.
- Make this a welcoming space.
- This is your time to slow down and enjoy.

---

80. Chozen Bays, *Mindful Eating*.

- Breathe.
- Remind yourself this present moment is safe.
- As you cook, notice the messages your body is communicating.
- Without judging, be interested. Lovingly observe.
- Be inquiring and continue to pull in breaths.
- Even notice how the food or cooking implements feel in your hands.
- As you sit and eat, allow yourself to experience the texture of food in your mouth.

Chewing Mantra

A mantra is an affirmation. It can be anything from a short phrase to a word that you repeat. Mantras are intended to reinforce support, calm, and love in the system. Many mantras are done during formal meditation or everyday acts. This mantra can be used while you nourish and befriend your body.

Repeat these five words in your head while you are chewing or preparing food:

Peace. Tranquility. Joy. Love. Gratitude.

Your Vagus Nerve

Remember that your vagus nerve works in service of your social well-being and safety.[81] Communal eating is one way to feel safe and connected, as coming together to eat can foster a deep sense of belonging.

When you are not feeling safe, you may rely on food to soothe you. If you are in a state of sympathetic mobility or dissociation,

---

81. Porges, *Polyvagal Safety*, 93.

it is important to first notice this. How many times have you eaten because you have not felt in your body, were depressed, or were emotionally overstimulated? In this way, you were using food to manage your affect. Those affects are deeply felt in the subdiaphragmatic nerves, as they are rooted in childhood attachment wounds and safety struggles.

Binge eating is a compensatory form of numbing or dissociation to manage uncomfortable affect in your system. When your stomach is painfully full, it is compelling those subdiaphragmatic nerves to create a sleepy disconnection. The nerves, the circulatory system, and everything required to digest food works overtime. Dorsal vagal engagement then slows you down to a sleepy crawl.

Food restriction or anorexia overstimulates sympathetic engagement. It takes a lot of fortitude to fight against one of your most primal needs that keeps you alive. Stressors from childhood that have already overstimulated your nervous system are then asked to stay in overdrive. IBS issues, obsessive rituals around food that you don't eat, and over exercising are all ways your nervous system is being asked to stay in hyper-arousal.

Your Chakras

The primal ways food brings comfort and soothing is felt deeply in the lower portions of your essential chakras. This is where the energy of early childhood attachment wounding is felt. During trauma processing it is not uncommon for clients to suddenly feel compelled or repelled to eat. They will put their hands on either their root, sacral, or solar plexus chakra.

While your chakric energy has the same resilient healing components as the rest of your body, eating disorders seem to take a hard toll on the etheric energy. Because of the beliefs around self-loathing, not feeling lovable, traumas, body image struggles, and boundary violations that created the resolute desires to restrict or binge, the etheric energy fields are particularly shut down.

During my time working in residential treatment with clients in their active eating disorders, clients' energy showed as chaotic or rigid. As one client told me, her anorexia was a bubble to the outside world that she refused to pop.

EXERCISE
Mindful Observing

Pay attention on purpose. Through utilizing sight, sound, taste, smell, and touch, let's get you applying those mindfulness skills during daily activities. This simply requires the intention to observe.

So often, you rush through life to the next thing: the next meeting, the next fitness goal, the next relationship. If you are in constant search outside of yourself to feel something wonderful, this is a gentle reminder to slow down. If you relax long enough to notice and connect to your body, it might become apparent that you rush so you don't have to feel. The desire to avoid the "feels" in our bodies drives a lot of unnecessary and self-destructive behaviors.

Observing your everyday tasks from a mindful perspective requires a few simple steps:

1. The intention to observe without judgment.
2. Connection to your breath
3. The ability to repeat steps 1 and 2.

Immediate Attention

Pay immediate attention to the object in front of you. If you are in a car hearing this, notice the taillights in the car in front of you. If you are in a room, then simply find an object right in front of you. Notice:

- How is the object shaped?
- What colors do you see?
- Is it one color or are there shades of that color?
- Observe it like you have never seen it before.
- Notice the shape.
- Notice the edges of the object.
- Notice any patterns.
- Notice the various ways the light is playing off the object.
- Now notice any thoughts you had around this process.
- Then redirect your attention back to the object you are noticing.

★ ★ ★

When you clutch on to that illusion of busy, you keep running harder and faster toward it. Eventually, the illusion you are hoping to grasp will dissipate, and you are left with how things are. There is great power in seeing things for what they are. This is where the power to change things lies. That power is always within yourself.

Katie's Story: Seeing Things for What She Wanted Them to Be

Katie came to me because she said she was depressed and anxious and had noticed her restrictive eating patterns were flaring. Katie was thirty-nine years old, an English professor at the local university, and never married. She claimed that marriage was all she ever wanted, yet it seemed to elude her. She worried that as she approached forty, she would never find her "happily ever after," as she put it.

"Tell me about your relationships," I said. "Are you seeing anyone now?"

Her "boyfriend," she explained, was twenty years older than her and living with another woman. "Charlie loves me. He's just needing some time to get his things together to move out."

"O-kay," I said. "How long has that been?"

Her eyes shifted away from mine. "It's been a few months."

"How long have you been dating?"

"About four months."

I nodded and was silent for a moment, waiting for her to fill in the rest of the story.

"This always happens, but Charlie loves me," she said. "We have spent every weekend together since we met."

"Hmmmm," I muttered. "Where's his girlfriend been during that time?"

She blushed. "Working."

"Do you think if he moves in with you he won't cheat on you?" I said. "A cheater is gonna cheat no matter who he's with."

She looked pale.

As I asked about her family history, she told me her parents have been married for forty years. It took Katie another session to admit the destructive dynamic both parents were in. It seemed her father was regularly unfaithful and would tell her mother about it. Then her parents would begin a destructive cycle that would pull the children into the cheating stories and raging. Her parents would end a few months of fighting and screaming with lurid make-up sex and going off on "second honeymoons."

"Yeah," Katie joked, "this is like their twentieth second honeymoon."

"Sounds like a nice drama cycle." I looked Katie in the eyes. "Do you think you repeat this cycle with emotionally unavailable men?"

"Mostly," she reported, she dated older married men. When I suggested she did this because she didn't really want to be in a relationship with someone emotionally available, she denied this.

"It would make sense," I suggested, "that you have conflicting feelings about marriage and commitment given what you saw growing up."

The following week Katie came in with a puffy face from crying. "Charlie broke up with me."

"I am sorry," I said.

"I should tell his girlfriend he was stepping out with me."

I sighed. "Can we work on what the driving force is behind all these married boyfriends instead of you lashing out to hurt his girlfriend?" I said.

We discussed Katie's family history in more detail. Because her father spent so much time outside of the house, Katie always felt abandoned by him. No matter what she did, she could not get his attention unless she took his side in her parents' fights.

"Geesh," she said. "No wonder I go for the old ones."

"Have you heard of the phrase 'what we are not aware of, we are bound to repeat'?" I said. "Do you want another man like this in your life?"

"I don't think I can go through this anymore," she said.

"Well, I can help you with that," I said. "Let's do some healing work for you, then see where the relationships go."

I started working with Katie's attachment struggles with her parents and how this formed her idea of what an adult relationship looked like. We worked through trauma issues using EMDR.

Katie started meditating to calm her mind. She said this was helping her desire to go long times without food. She was working on not trying to control things she could control, such as her eating patterns, because of all the other things and people in her life she could not control.

We agreed that she would not date for a few months. We also discussed that when she decided to date again, we would work through what kind of qualities she might want in a person to date first.

"Like an actually single one that isn't my father's age?" she joked.

"Good start."

Katie did eventually start dating, with many perimeters in place. Aside from having men who were not committed to other women on her checklist, we broke down what emotional availability looked like—not only in them but herself. With a deliberately slow approach, Katie found a man that was her age and available.

"I'm really trying to see things for what they are," she said, "not what I want them to be."

We worked with her experiences of avoidance when they would creep in. She was learning to set boundaries with others and know what boundaries looked like within herself. She also set limits with her parents and refused to discuss anything about their marriage with them.

Eventually, after two years of dating the same man, she got engaged. She still sees me when she feels the urge to run, but she reports that she enjoys being in an actual relationship with someone she can know for who he is and not a replacement for an unavailable father.

EXERCISE
Vipassana Meditation

Vipassana meditation is intended to provide insight. Insight meditation is the practice of being aware of sensations, which will lead to the true nature of existence. In Pali, the word *Vipassana* means "special seeing." It means to see things as they really are. Bringing understanding to the mind and heart takes inquiry and non-judgment.[82] This leave space to see your truth.

You don't have to sit in a perfect lotus position to formally meditate. You can find a chair, cushion, or whatever allows you to feel settled and safe. The only major requirement is to know that you have a sacred, safe room or place to sit. You can even find a shawl if you believe you will get cold. Know where you can find your spot, and return to it as you develop confidence in just sitting.

Like all things that are simple in nature, the results are profound and take time to cultivate. To develop a mastery over "non-doing" takes patience. Repetition builds upon itself. Make time each day to meditate. Start with a few minutes and increase time gradually. Don't set yourself up to fail by starting

---

82. Goldstein and Kornfield, *Seeking the Heart of Wisdom*, 81.

out meditating for a long period of time. Set a timer on your phone so you can relax into the process and not worry about watching the clock.

- As you sit, keep your spine straight but not taut. This helps you stay connected to your body and be present yet still.
- Rest your arms on your thighs.
- If you are sitting in a chair, keep your feet on the floor.
- If you are sitting on a cushion, make sure your hips are more elevated than your knees.
- If your knees will be on the ground, consider how you are sitting as a triangle, with the bottom squares of your knees balancing the body with the spine long.
- Now, just follow your breath.
- Notice the sensations of your breath as they come in through your nose and down the back of your throat.
- Continue to trace the path of your breath
- Be curious and observant.
- Notice the breath as it pulls into your lungs.
- Follow the breath out through your throat and nostrils.
- Be curious about any affect in your body.
- Breathe and stay curious.
- When your mind wanders, because it will, just return to your breath.

If a mantra helps to keep you focused and centered, try this one:

I am Peace.

I am Joy.

I am Love.

I am Gratitude.

As with any new practice, meditation will help build structure for you over time. Soon, those first few minutes will become ten, twenty, or even thirty.

Summary

Mindfulness comes from the ancient Hindu practices in the Pali tradition. Pali was one of the languages of the ancient Buddhist scriptures. In Pali, the word *Vipassana* means "special seeing." Western-centered mindfulness practices have been incorporated into many healing modalities, from therapy to addiction recovery to stress reduction by various American Buddhist educators.

Through awareness of thoughts and the breath and inquiring, you can gauge your neuroception. Noticing the energy flow in your body, which also includes the etheric energies in your chakras, takes awareness and curiosity. This can be done as you stay present and non-judgmental to yourself and the situations around you.

There are many ways to apply mindfulness in your everyday life, from walking to listening to eating. Being present while engaging in all activities, not just formal Vipassana meditation, allows you the only kind of control you actually possess, which is power over how you choose to express yourself.

CHAPTER 6

WHAT HAPPENS IN VAGUS STAYS IN VAGUS—IF YOU'RE NOT CAREFUL

•————————•

How easily your nervous system bounces back from stressors is called vagal tone.[83] This is a way to gauge vagus nerve health. Having a healthy nervous system makes a world of difference, as it not only reads your life situations but sustains your respiratory, circulatory, and digestive systems. When your body is in balance, you can manage life with more equanimity. Equanimity is the crux of being mindful and staying calm.

You turn lights on in your house every night. I'm guessing you rarely consider the electrical wiring and perhaps the condition it's in. Using this metaphor, consider the vagus nerve is your wiring that keeps things well lit at home.

The health of your body is the health of your vagus.[84] Cardiovascular workouts are vagus nerve workouts. Making dietary changes for managing inflammation and gut health is managing vagus nerve health. Yoga brings flexibly to the spine, which is vagus nerve health.[85]

As you age, everything gets a little more worn: your joints, your skin, and even your nervous system. You work out to keep

---

83. Porges, *Polyvagal Safety*, 42.
84. Rosenberg, *Accessing the Healing Power of the Vagus Nerve*.
85. Schwartz, *Applied Polyvagal Theory in Yoga*.

your heart, lungs, and muscles strong, but do you realize you are serving your nervous system? After all, what manages the breathing of those lungs and the beating of your heart? Because your vagus nerve is the main channel to and from the major organs that your cardiologist, pulmonologist, gastroenterologist, nephrologist, urologist, and otolaryngologist tend to, when you care for these parts of your body, you are caring for your vagus nerve health too.

When the lights don't come on in your house, the first thing you look at is the circuitry. If the electricity works, life continues with a sense of comfort. If it doesn't, life gets hard very fast. Suddenly, your breathing is disrupted. The rhythm of your heart and blood pressure become irregular. Your mood is affected, your digestion is bad, and your thinking is off.

When your vagus nerve is not functioning optimally, you experience bloating and stomach upset that includes diarrhea, constipation, reflux, or struggles with swallowing. Food stops moving or moves too fast through your system. You can develop sleep and fatigue issues, dizziness, or fainting spells. Inflammation occurs.[86] Shingles is an example of a viral load that courses along the nervous system; so are meningitis and encephalitis.[87] You have multiple immune barriers that can protect your nervous system. However, the blood can also carry many viruses that infect the tissue of the nervous system.

The following is a quick survey to give you an indication of your vagus nerve health. Like many health-related factors, there are some things you can change by modifying behaviors. Other aspects of your health have to be managed. Befriending your body is the best first step.

---

86. Rosenberg, *Accessing the Healing Power of the Vagus Nerve*, 2–6.
87. Koyuncu et al., "Virus Infections in the Nervous System."

EXERCISE
Checking In with Your Vagus Nerve Health

This is a general survey for you to get an idea of your vagal tone:

Do you want to take naps but cannot seem to sleep?

Yes   No

Do you struggle to fall asleep at night even though you're tired?

Yes   No

Do you have a hard time getting up in the morning?

Yes   No

Do you struggle getting out of bed at all?

Yes   No

Is it hard for you to feel calm even when you try to be?

Yes   No

Do you struggle with regular diarrhea?

Yes   No

Do you struggle with regular constipation?

Yes   No

Do you faint for inexplicable reasons?

Yes   No

Do you have problems swallowing food?

Yes   No

Do you have heartburn issues?

Yes   No

Do you have diabetes or are prediabetic?

Yes   No

Do you struggle with inflammation?

Yes   No

When something shocking happens, do you regain calm easily?

Yes   No

If something scary happens, do you dissociate easily?

Yes   No

Have you had childhood trauma?

Yes   No

If there are more yes answers from this questionnaire than no answers, then you might struggle with your vagal tone. This is a good way to get you thinking about your nervous system health and is intended to empower you to heal. Information is empowering. If you are struggling, then you can identify the solutions. Do not fret; we all have issues with vagal tone at one point or another in our lives.

Indicators of Vagus Nerve Problems

Before you can find a solution, you have to understand the problem. Let's look at some things that are problematic or indicators of potentially larger issues. Remember, the vagus nerve connects to all the major organs in your body. If you are struggling with the health of a major organ, there is a chance the autonomic nerves that connect to that organ need attention as well.

Fainting

Many people have come up to me after I have spoken about the vagus nerve and chakras. Some have told me stories about how they faint when they are exposed to certain events or stimuli. They say their doctors have not found any major health problems but have told them they experience something called vasovagal syncope. *Syncope* means fainting.

This happens when the nerves to your heart get overstimulated and you have a sudden loss of blood to the brain. Heat, stress, physical pain, traumatic situations that stress the system, or even hunger can arouse this response. Medical procedures (or the thought of them), the sight of needles, fear of harm or blood, and certainly having your blood drawn can do this.[88] Even pressing down too hard during a bowel movement can create a fainting spell. This is a stress reaction that induces a medical problem.

Vasovagal syncope is an immediate response in your nervous system. Many people are waking up before they understand what even happened to them. I know one person who stepped on a branch while hiking. That branch flipped up and hit the side of that person's neck. They passed out briefly. That slap to the jugular dropped blood pressure in that person's system. Other than a slight bruise, they were fine (and got checked by a doctor afterward).

When you get overtired or exhausted do you faint? Standing too long, especially with your knees locked, can do this. I was once at a high school Christmas choir performance. Suddenly, half the

---

88. "Vasovagal Syncope."

choir, one by one, dropped down behind the balustrade and out of sight. The performance had to be stopped while the choir director reminded the students to unlock their knees. Everyone was fine, the concert resumed, and there was lot of nervous laughter about it afterward.

The general medical explanation for vasovagal syncope is that your blood pressure drops quickly because of a rapid sympathetic response from your vagus nerve. This usually happens when standing or sitting.

When a person faints as a result of vasovagal syncope, they may look like they are having a seizure.[89] They may experience a narrowed field of vision or a flushed feeling before fainting. Their eyes may roll back, and they have a weak pulse. Recovery time is rapid; however, there is a risk of fainting again. Being cautious about how to care for themselves afterward is important. Lying down with feet propped up or putting their head between their knees will help bring the blood flow back to the brain.

If you have had this happen and have not had a diagnosis, please don't diagnose yourself based on this information. Talk to your doctor to rule out anything more serious. Fainting can be an indicator of more serious issues. Following an episode, it is important to slow down and lie down if possible, until your system can regulate. Drinking liquids with electrolytes and making sure you have food in your stomach will be helpful. Just pace yourself a bit and take good care.

---

89. Aydin et al., "Management and Therapy of Vasovagal Syncope," 308–15.

Trauma Responses that May
Cause Vasovagal Syncope

Perhaps you experienced a moment in childhood that was over-whelming and you don't remember it. Now every time you are in this situation you faint. This might not make sense to you as an adult, but your body is remembering this through neuroception.[90]

One client of mine wanted to take up horseback riding but stated every time she attempted to mount the horse she would faint. She had to stop riding, which was really disappointing to her since she loved horses.

When she asked her mother if there was anything in her past that had to do with horses, the family could not think of anything. A while later, her older brother reminded her of a time when she was two years old. She slid onto the back of a neighbor's Great Dane, and the dog ran, throwing my client across the room. She hit her head and was knocked out for a short time.

This seemed along the lines of the work I could help her with and not out of my scope of practice, so, through the protocols of EMDR, we alleviated her body's dorsal vagal fear response that registered danger when she sat on the back of an animal. After clearing the trauma from her system, she was able to start riding again, as her system was no longer registering threat.

* * *

There are two medically induced forms of vasovagal syncope. One is common in men over fifty. This is called carotid sinus syndrome. It occurs when pressure is applied to the neck and has happened

---

90. Porges, *The Polyvagal Theory*, 194.

to men while shaving, wearing tight neck collars, or turning their neck a certain way.

The second is called situational syncope. It's a reflex that happens when coughing, during bowel movements, after a meal, or when swallowing. While these are not commonly life-threatening, fainting in itself can cause big problems—especially near ceramic or porcelain bathroom fixtures. Again, get checked out by a medical professional to rule out more serious conditions if you experience this.

Gastroparesis

When the vagus nerve is damaged and the gut-brain axis does not function properly, this can stop food from easily moving into your intestines from your stomach.[91] Dehydration, constipation, fatigue, and infection can occur with gastropareses.

Gastroparesis happens when the stomach muscles fail to contract and efficiently move food into the small intestines. This occurs because of damage to the vagus, which signals this process. The nerve cannot innervate strongly enough to contract the stomach. Food can sit too long in the stomach then, and your digestive process slows. For some, digestion hurts, and over time the body does not absorb the nutrients it needs. If all the food is not processed through the stomach, a hardened mass called a bezoar can develop. This happens in both humans and animals.

There are a few different types of gastropareses. One is diabetes related. The nerve fibers become damaged from high blood glucose. This wears down the myelinated sheath that coats the nerves. Remember that your ventral vagal fibers are myelinated,

---

91. Hui and Page, "Altered Vagal Signaling and Its Pathophysiological Roles in Functional Dyspepsia."

which helps information flow faster. Over time, the brain, heart, lungs, and all supradiaphragmatic functions slow.

According to the National Institutes of Health, 11.3 percent of the population in the United States has diabetes. Diabetes is the single most cause for gastroparesis and accounts for about a third of the cases. Roughly 50 percent of diabetic patients have trouble with digestion and aren't aware of it. As diabetes develops, the nerve fibers lose their ability to innervate and send signals to the organs.[92]

Another form of gastroparesis may be a complication from surgery. This may cause pinched nerves along the vagus nerve. Intubation or prolonged ventilation are two ways this may happen. Throat or neck surgery are another. Pinched cranial nerves can cause stomach upset or slow the innervation of the nerves.

Idiopathic gastroparesis occurs for no medically identifiable reason. Idiopathic gastroparesis is the second most commonly occurring digestive issue and can stump patients and medical staff.[93] Gastroparesis feels like all the symptoms mentioned earlier: bloating, gaseousness, nauseousness, stomach pain, or reflux. The pain varies from person to person and some people who experience higher levels of pain may have sensitized nerve fibers. When the food does eventually pass, you may see pieces of undigested food in the toilet. This is a condition that needs to be looked at by a medical doctor with a plan put in place. However, it is manageable with long-term, intentional, holistic care.

92. "Diabetes Statistics."
93. Parkman, "Idiopathic Gastroparesis," 59–68.

Fatigue

Fatigue is a nondescript, gloomy experience. You look fine to others, but you are not feeling fine. It's hard to get any affirmation from people about your experience because it's hard to see that you do not feel well, and they may just think you're lazy or unwilling to help. I describe fatigue to my clients as being exhausted from the inside out, not the normal outside-in tired that someone feels at the end of a busy day. This is because your "insides" are exhausted.

One of the reasons people struggle with fatigue is that the vagus nerve modulates the hypothalamic-pituitary-adrenal axis (HPA). As mentioned, this axis regulates so much, including your fight-or-flight (sympathetic) responses. When you are under constant threat of harm, your sympathetic branch of the vagus nerve listens to the cues of the brain and fires off all the messages the body needs to keep itself safe. It does this by sending signals to the adrenal glands to release cortisol into your bloodstream. This cortisol is designed to move you into action. It sends signals to the heart to beat faster as the muscles constrict in an attempt to run or fight off an offender. Over time, if you do not find ways to restabilize the system, you expend cortisol to the point that the system doesn't work optimally.[94] Our adrenal glands then produce less of this hormone, and we eventually develop adrenal fatigue symptoms.

When a child grows up in an environment where they are under constant threat, their sympathetic branch is on overdrive. This constant stimulation wears down the HPA axis over time, and the individual may require medicines in adulthood that decrease

---

94. Wilson, *Adrenal Fatigue*, 50.

hyperarousal.[95] If this persists without any restoration to the system, the adrenals deplete. This is called Addison's disease. Given that the adrenals also produce important hormones that affect sex drive and mood, these little glands on the top of your kidneys are vital to all aspects of your life.

One of the other jobs of cortisol is to set your diurnal patterns. Cortisol levels are higher in the morning and lower at night so you can sleep. When your cortisol is depleted, you have the opposite experience: slow mornings and awake nights. Sleep is not quality, even though you might imagine with fatigue you would be exhausted and sleep deeply. This can be a sign that you're experiencing fatigue from long-term overactivation of the HPA axis.

There are many situations where people are under constant, long-term threat. Living in war-torn countries, poverty-stricken places, or racially minimized areas are all examples. People who are in constant danger of survival struggle with major health issues, and those such as ICU and ER medical staff, first responders, and police officers have to work hard to manage their physical and emotional health on the off-hours. Their workdays require the constant vigilance of keeping their systems in a present but sympathetic state.

Keeping a balance in your daily routine that alleviates unnecessary stressors is one way to manage your system. Walking, quietly sitting, laughing with friends, and engaging in mindful meditation are some ways. Hiking or sitting in nature can replete your system as well. This is because you are bringing safety cues back into your system.

What do your days look like? Are there times you can be more intentional and caring for yourself. How are you doing this?

---

95. Van der Kolk, *The Body Keeps the Score*, 227.

Exercising Too Much

This is an interesting one since regular exercise is vital to the health of every aspect of your body, including your vagus nerve. However, excessive exercise, especially if you are struggling with fatigue issues, can drain your adrenal glands instead of fortifying them. I had to learn this one the hard way when I was in grad school, stressed and suddenly struggling with long distances on my road bike.

Overtraining syndrome (OS) can deplete the adrenals and cause an imbalance of hormones in your system.[96] Many triathletes struggle with this. The training isn't the problem in itself. When your body is put under undue strain for long periods of time and you also train heavily, this can create adrenal insufficiency. I personally had to ride shorter distances and slower when I discovered my body was fatigued from graduate school demands. To be honest, I had never even heard of adrenal fatigue back in the early 2000s. It took a doctor friend who was practicing "boutique" medicine to take a saliva test from me. This was the only way to get a measurement of the amount of cortisol I was producing throughout the day. When he told me the results showed I had almost no cortisol, back then, I had no idea what he meant. However, that did lead me into some helpful research not only for me but for my clients.

My personal journey of adrenal repair led me to an awareness of why my clients struggle with fatigue. The good news is that adrenals, if treated well, will rebuild over time, but attention to your stress levels will always be imperative.

---

96. Brooks and Carter, "Overtraining, Exercise, and Adrenal Insufficiency."

Alcohol

Have you ever felt irritable and short-tempered after a night on the town? Has your thinking been foggy and your body tired after too much drinking? "Frayed nerves" are a symptom of an overuse of alcohol in your system.

We talk about people who die of cirrhosis of the liver from heavy drinking. Much is discussed about alcohol's effects on the liver, kidneys, and digestive tract, not to mention the heart, arteries, and brain. We almost never discuss someone's death from dysfunction of the vagus nerve due to alcoholism.[97] Yet, our nervous system atrophies over time from heavy alcohol use.

The effects of heavy drinking on the nervous system and vagus nerve can be severe.[98] The central nervous system is the conduit to all other systems and organs in the body. It carries alcohol along the membrane fibers. Alcohol crosses these membrane barriers and rapidly infuses into your body. It immediately slows down your cognition because it interferes with the receptors in your brain and contracts brain tissue. Speech becomes halting. Thoughts jumble. The body losses its proprioception.

A few drinks after work feel immediately calming because they suppress the excitatory nerves along your neuronal pathways. If a few drinks regularly becomes a night on the town, you are repatterning the communication pathways in your body. Your system becomes dependent on this outer source for calming. When you realize the vagus nerve is the major connector to your major organs, which process and digest ethanol, you can see how your nervous system is experiencing the same damage as those organs.

---

97. Guo et al., "Pathological Changes in the Vagus Nerve in Diabetes and Chronic Alcoholism."
98. Mukherjee, "Alcoholism and Its Effects on the Central Nervous System."

Also, the more you drink, the more risk of inflammation you can experience. Alcohol is, after all, a form of sugar and challenges your whole system to digest. Over time alcohol creates what is known as alcoholic neuropathy. Neuropathy is a numbness, pain, or weakness of the nerves.

Hoarseness in your voice can be an indicator that the nervous system is experiencing strain, so can something called dysphagia, which is an impairment of speech.[99] While hoarseness of the voice can also occur with other injuries to the nervous system, we can immediately notice this during a hangover. Like all things, a middle way is encouraged, even when drinking. Notice how the things you consume affect your body; this helps you stay in balance.

Sugar

Glucose is a major energy source for the nervous system. Your brain and nervous system and all organs have a finely tuned structure in place to process glucose. The nervous system and brain make up a major portion of the systems that need this glucose.

Your body breaks down the sugary sweets you eat into glucose. However, too much of a sugary diet can impair the nervous system. This slows down cognitive functioning and can start a loop of needing more sugar. Excess amounts of sugar force your body into overdrive to keep blood glucose levels managed. Inflammation kicks in, and the myelin sheath experiences oxidative stress, which damages cells and tissue. Too much sugar sets off an imbalance in your system that can leave you fatigued, which affects mood and overall energy levels.

---

99. Novak and Victor, "The Vagus and Sympathetic Nerves in Alcoholic Poly-neuropathy," 273–84.

Childhood Abuse

Like anything that receives long-term wear and tear, the vagus nerve can decrease in efficacy when the sympathetic branch is constantly overstimulated. This is particularly at play with adult survivors of childhood abuse.[100] Bouncing back from stressors gets harder. Irritability and exhaustion become the norm.

Some of the ways the vagus nerve loses its neuroplasticity are organic. Some are from long-term emotional stressors to the body. As a trauma therapist, I see clients who grew up in families that were chaotic, rageful, and unsafe. Sometimes that lack of safety is confusing because there may not have been any physical or sexual abuse, which is what so many people think of when they hear the word *abuse*. There may not have even been financial or educational limits on resources, which confuses others, as childhood abuse is unduly associated only with stressors of poverty. However, any time a child is forced into unsafe situations—emotionally or physically—generates a sympathetic response in their system. Over time, those neurobiological reactions are the norm.

Even if the parents regularly argue in front of the child, if the child is asked to perform tasks they are not developmentally capable of but fear being "in trouble" for, or even if the child is expected to meet the grown-ups' emotional needs, this creates a lack of well-being. Absent or enmeshed parents can create anxiety, as the child struggles with emotional and psychological boundaries and will not know how to apply them in adulthood.

As the child grows, they become programmed to be on high alert or shut down. They develop coping strategies to manage situations they might believe are just normal. Hypervigilance or

---

100. Fisher, *Healing the Fragmented Selves of Trauma Survivors*, 127.

dissociation might be how the child gets through life. Disordered eating or other addictive behaviors begin as a way to manage feeling overstimulated.

One of the first things I ask a client as I am learning their history is if they experience a constant, inexplicable achiness in their mid-upper back along the top of their kidneys. They all say yes. We discuss any gastrointestinal issues or fatigue. This is where the education about their nervous system, the physical effects of their trauma, and ways to find caring resources begins.

Since my grad school days, much research around the HPA axis, constant sympathetic arousal, and adrenal fatigue has been published. Becoming trauma informed about your own body's reactions is a starting point for healing. To clear trauma from your system, particularly to develop neuroplasticity in the brain and the vagus nerve, requires a level of trust and connection to your body. Incorporating safety into your life through multiple levels of self-care is a solid step.

Organic Issues

Organic issues are things inside your body that affect the functioning of the vagus nerve. Some of the major damage to the vagus nerve can come from viruses.[101] A virus, such as herpes simplex virus (HSV-1 and HSV-2), can impair the cells of the nerve fibers. Once your body contracts the herpes simplex virus, it is stored and can on occasion flare up. HSV-1 is what we understand to be cold sores, which generally present on the lips or face. HSV-2 is genital herpes.

---

101. Bello-Morales et al., "The Role of Herpes Simplex Virus Type 1 Infection in Demyelination of the Central Nervous System."

While these viruses are contracted through skin-to-skin contact, they travel to an area of the brain where they can lie dormant. The virus then stores in a cranial nerve ganglion called the trigeminal ganglion. The viruses can flare up during times of stress.

The same holds true for the varicella-zoster virus, which is the virus that causes chicken pox. Once (generally) a child has contracted the virus, the virus travels through the bloodstream and settles in the dorsal ganglion of the vagus nerve. When the body is under large amounts of stress, the virus resurfaces along infected nerve fibers and creates a stinging, tingling sensation along the skin. Eventually, the skin blisters in the same pocked way it did when experiencing chicken pox.

Many studies are being conducted about the long-term effects of SARS-CoV-2 and how the virus stores in the cranial nerves.[102] Studies are also being conducted to explore possible routes of pathogens into the brain via the vagus nerve, as it is the largest of the cranial nerves.

Learning about neurodegenerative diseases and how they affect mental health is vital. Parkinson's is one of those diseases that can store in the nervous system and make its way to the brain, affecting neuronal functioning through muscle weakness and shaking. There is also research suggesting that Parkinson's might start in the gut and make its way along the vagus neuronal pathways.[103]

Bacterial infections can inflame the vagus nerve and affect brain function. Gut health is usually a key to how well your nervous system is functioning. The gut-brain axis is very complex and

---

102. Taha et al., "Effects of Non-Invasive Vagus Nerve Stimulation on Inflammatory Markers in COVID-19 Patients."

103. "New Evidence Suggests Link Between Gut Health and Parkinson's Disease."

something to be taken seriously.[104] Microbiota transfer information from the gastrointestinal tract up to the brain. If you're struggling with dietary issues and weight issues, you are more susceptible to inflammation.

Stinking Thinking

Your mind is geared to seek out danger; it's that negative bias we've been talking about. It's the ancient programing that kept your ancestors alive. With sight, smell, and hearing, your nervous system is looking for things that might harm you. How much you focus on the negative is reflected in how your brain prioritizes things.

So, the question is: How and what do you think? How stinking are your thought patterns?

If you are not aware that you can look at things differently, then you are bound to repeat whatever patterns have been set.[105] Apply discernment. Challenge what upsets you. What shocks you may be an illusion, but your vagus nerve, your brain, and all the organs it communicates with don't know that.

Over time, these thoughts in the form of neurotransmitters deepen the groove of pathways in your mind. These pathways get set, and soon you are deeper in the illusion than you realize. The messages from your brain are sent down to the nervous system in a split second, and before you realize what is happening your neuroception is registering menace. Sounds exhausting, doesn't it? Mindful curiosity of how your thoughts fire signals in your body is the way forward.[106]

---

104. Mayer, *The Mind-Gut Connection*, 22.
105. Beck, *Cognitive Behavioral Therapy*.
106. Kabat-Zinn, *Full Catastrophe Living*.

Unsafe People

We are not meant to be disconnected from others. We need community; having community is another evolutionary process that kept our species going.[107] Caring community keeps you safe.

How you interact with others can be a spiritual experience with much fulfilment and growth for you. Alleviating judgment and listening in a different way can connect you to the light of the person or people you are with—and bring out the light within you.

However, there are unsafe people in the world and not just physically violent ones. We can also be around emotionally and psychologically unsafe ones. Listening to how your body feels around people is key. Are you depleted when you are with them? Does what they say not match up with what they do? Are they attempting to frame you as a certain kind of person when you know you are not that way? These may be gaslighting tactics.

Just notice the experience of connection or disruption in your body and be honest with how this feels. Don't doubt your internal experience.

Relating to unsafe people might even include people you think should be safe, such as a partner, spouse, friend, or family member. If you have grown up in a household that sent mixed messages of safety, you might have mixed messages of who is safe in adulthood. Your brain and nervous system might register confusion because these unsafe people feel familiar. Your neuroception becomes faulty and misreads social cues. This is where a mindful, slower approach can help you center in the truth of your being.

Below is an example of a client that did not understand the emotional components that affected the health of her vagus nerve.

---

107. Porges, *Polyvagal Safety*, 27.

She did everything to tone her body and eat right, but she was unaware of how the people in her life were making her sick.

Kai's Story: How Her Vagus Didn't Serve Her Because She Didn't Serve It

Kai was a kinesiology researcher at a major university. She came to me because of high levels of anxiety that felt so out of control when she wasn't working or working out that she had developed an abuse of alcohol. Kai had a raspy voice and was always dressed in expensive leggings and workout tops. Even when showered and in full makeup, she wore her workout wear. Her blonde hair was always brushed and managed. She was aware of the stunning image she projected when she passed by people. As she referred to her sexuality, she at once "put it out there" and was repelled by it.

Her marriage was in trouble since Kai was unable—or as she said, unwilling—to have sex without a lot of wine in her system. Because work was a place where she could channel her anxiety and working out daily at the campus gym seemed to "blow off steam" for her, she was coming home later and later. She told me that her husband felt he was being ignored.

"I know I'm not spending enough time at home, but frankly, he's starting to annoy me." Kai's voice was deep and had a strained tone to it.

"Can you tell me more?"

She shrugged and ran her hands through her hair. "Everyone is starting to annoy me, really."

Kai was working out several times a day, including leading some spinning classes.

She would have a drink with friends before she went home and always had a least one or two glasses with dinner. The more she was drinking, the more agitated she would get. Her mother wasn't helping the situation either, according to Kai. Her mother regularly asked Kai to participate in complaining about family members, including her father and Kai's own husband.

The more Kai spoke, the raspier her voice got. Through the weeks in therapy with me, her voice was cracking, and she had to regularly clear her throat. She complained one day that her focus was completely "shot" at work. She blamed it on her husband, even though he wasn't demanding much of her time anymore. Kai also said she could not sleep.

"I'm going to be frank," I finally said one day. "I think your high levels of stress have produced deficiencies in your autonomic nervous system. Certainly your regular drinking and overexercising has too. You sound like you're in for some major health issues."

I explained to Kai that through excessive working out and regular drinking, along with a regular dose of negativity and gossip from her mother, she was depleting her vagus nerve. "Your regular gossiping might feel good in the moment, but it's unnecessarily plucking at your sympathetic nervous system. Even your voice is getting hoarse, which tells me it might be affecting your vocal cords. Do you have stomach issues?"

Kai's mouth dropped open, and she stared a moment. "How do I not know this?"

I told her what I had learned around the vagus nerve in regards to trauma processing and how a healthy nervous system was vital to calm. This got her listening, especially given her focus was on health-related things. We discussed how excessive working out might actually be depleting her adrenals and cortisol, which also affects her sex hormones.

"Let's start by setting some limits around your mom," I said.

Kai looked nervous. "Not sure I can do that."

We discussed how her mother was using Kai as an emotional spouse and didn't honor Kai's boundaries. Her mother would gripe about her father to Kai, which made Kai feel sick. Once Kai married, her mother's calls to her intensified.

Kai managed feelings of enmeshment with her mother by long-distance cycling and running and wine. Now that she was married and mother was calling more, she was feeling smothered but afraid to admit that to herself. Fearing she was not being a good daughter, she was in turn terrified about being a good wife.

Co-regulation was not "safe" for Kai because it wasn't co-regulation; it was constant bombardment of boundaries. Kai learned to regulate her own system by running. The more people put demands on her affections, the more she worked out.

"What's the hardest part of setting limits with your mom?"

"Well." She gave me an uncomfortable smile, and her face reddened. "She's pretty overwhelming. She doesn't take no for an answer easily. She might even start gossiping about me."

"Do you think she's doing that anyway?"

"Yeah," she said. "She always does, but I think I was hoping if I joined in she wouldn't talk so badly about me. She's really kind of heinous."

"Some people will never change no matter how hard we try," I said. "You said she calls about four times a day when you're at work, right?"

She nodded.

"So, maybe at first you use work as the reason you don't pick up the phone. That's an easy boundary."

"Oh, lord." Kai slumped in the chair and looked like a young teenager who was about to get a punishment for acting out. "She would probably show up at the building."

"Is that a fear or a reality?"

Kai was silent for a minute and bit her lower lip. "Well, she's never actually done it." She looked up at me. "She did do that in college once and showed up at my dorm one night when I wasn't answering my phone."

"Wow. That wasn't embarrassing, was it?" I joked.

"It was awful."

"However, she doesn't have that kind of power over you now," I said. "Unless you give it to her."

I could see Kai running the scenario of her mother showing up at the research center. "She wouldn't make it past security." Kai giggled.

"She sounds like a woman that's afraid to lose perceived power over people."

"Hmmmm." Kai nodded. "I hadn't thought of that before."

"Those people don't really have much power anyway," I said. "If you were to tell her what the phone call boundaries were, what would you want to say?"

"Don't call me at work anymore. It's affecting my performance." Kai seemed pleased with that. "It's not a lie."

"Okay," I said. "Let's start there."

The next week Kai came in laughing. "It worked."

"How do you feel?"

"Lighter," she said. "Now let's work on limiting phone calls after hours."

Kai discovered that despite some pushback her mother honored her limits. This gave Kai a sense of independence she probably never felt with her mother before. I suggested that Kai and her husband do some marriage counseling to reset limits and expectations in the marriage. That seemed to work.

"We're having sex more," she laughed. "Weirdly, I'm also going to the gym less and I feel better."

EXERCISE
Blowing Off Steam

If we observe children and their natural habits more, we can see great examples of how to live intuitively in our own bodies. Play and impulsive moments of skipping, jumping, rolling, and stretching are so natural to children—so is using their voice.

This exercise will require some children's toys. Get some balloons, bubbles, whistles, or any toys that require blowing. Then just play with them. If you struggle with blowing up any balloons, see if you can improve this over time. You will be developing your lung capacity and improving vagal tone.

What Any of This Has to Do with the Soul

The chakras and auras are the energies that can be sensed but not normally seen by the naked eye. This is Soul energy that emanates beyond the body. When your body struggles with the pain or illness of past traumas, that suffering courses your biology. It reveals itself in the physical systems we just talked about. Since your body acts as the gatekeeper to Soul energy expressed outward, your human pain mixes with your etheric field and can be felt before your physical self walks in the room.

Energy healers approach healing from the direction of clearing these fields. Trauma therapists approach this from the clearing of traumatic patterns and reintegrating safety in the nervous system. The more you can "undo" the old pain and reestablish patterns that sustain growth and safety, the more you can access the higher, wiser energy of Soul.

Like attracts like. Frequency attracts frequency.[108] The wounded addict draws to them other addicts. The rage-filled controller attracts the submissive tolerator of the rage. While it may appear that people with these wounded aspects actually pull in others to engage, the other people with their wounds might be like a Venn diagram or a yin yang symbol of puzzle pieces. For instance, while someone who identifies as an addict might not marry someone that uses drugs, the person they are in relationship with might have a level of tolerance for that addiction. Their interplay just looks different and facilitates the wounded dance of childhood.

We are drawn to connect. If we can't do it in love and boundaries, we will do it through a compulsive, familiar, repetitive dance. Any energy worker will tell you they see these energies in both the chakras and the auric field. What they intuit is coming from the denser experience of your internal wiring system and is casting shadows outward. The wounds are an extension of what the vagus nerve and your organs are holding, and they expose themselves outward.

It is not just in similar woundedness that we connect. We are drawn through similarities such as love, preferences, and sound. How much we heal physically and psychologically also reveals itself in the energy that is projected outward from our corporal bodies.

Summary

Having a healthy nervous system is vital to accurately reading your life situations. The health of the vagus nerve provides a sustainability to your whole system. When your body is in balance,

---

108. Peirce, *Frequency*.

you can manage everything with more equanimity. Some indicators that your vagus nerve health may not be optimal are fatigue, organic issues such as viruses and bacterial infections, gastroparesis, effects of trauma, poor diet, inflammation, alcohol abuse, and even the way you think, since this creates anxiety and experiences of lack of safety in your system.

When your body struggles, when it holds on to energies of pain or illness, it reveals this through the less dense energies of the chakras and auric field. The wounds are an extension of what the vagus nerve and your organs are holding, and they expose themselves outward. This creates a denser barrier for your internal light of Soul to shine beyond. Being mindful of how your body is functioning can help you discern health issues, provide awareness of what your needs are so you can heal, and lead with your higher, wiser light.

CHAPTER 7
A HEALTHY NERVOUS SYSTEM IS A MINDFUL NERVOUS SYSTEM

N ow that we've discussed some problems related to vagus nerve health, let's discuss some solutions to facilitate the healing of your physical body. I can't express enough that applying a curious, nonjudgmental approach to your physical and emotional state is the first step to understanding what your nervous system health is telling you. Old habits can die hard. Be inquisitive and trust you will ultimately know what's right for you. Your internal light is always safe and holds your truth. Centering and breathing to access it through your body changes everything.

Make changes that you can maintain. Don't take massive leaps; just do what feels right for you. Sometimes the health challenges are big and we are forced to make extreme turnarounds in our behaviors and habits. Many times we can get proactive and incorporate small things that lead to major outcomes.

Remember that your nervous system, like all other parts of your body, is neutral. In other words, it is responding to what you put into it. Your body is just doing what you are asking it to do. It is the applied meaning you put to your body in general that signals how your body does its job.

By instilling calm and safety, your system will feel calm and safe. By instilling fear and hatred, your system will activate in fear and hatred. Sounds simple but you would be surprised how hard old patterns are to break—especially if you don't see them.

If you have been taught your body is the enemy, it will respond accordingly because you have trained it to backfire on you. Your body is here in service of you. Be curious about your mental health. This will affect your physical health, and you will find the best solutions.

Your body does not lie. You just have to be open to the idea that your body holds the ultimate truth and that if you listen in a compassionate way, you will find true answers. If you are uncertain about how to proceed in a situation, then settle and listen to what your body says. If you are afraid, check in with your body. It will show you the way, and you will find calm. Your body will even give you answers to its own healing—if you listen.

Consider that you are in a collaborative relationship with your body. When you collaborate with other people, do you share ideas and listen to theirs for a greater outcome for all? Or do you attempt to control the dynamic until you get your way? Are you present to hear new concepts? Or do you shout other people down? Are you focused on an effective outcome, or do you want to seek contrary results?

Let's explore these questions with the following exercise. It will help you attune to the chakras and the vagus nerve through full body collaboration. I have done this with my clients and myself. If you have never asked your body to be your confidant and your guide, I think you will be pleasantly surprised at the outcome. You can take your time with this. If you need to do a chakra a day, do that. If you want to try each chakra at once, do that. Go at your own pace, and since you might have not done something like this before, it will take time to know what your pace is. As you grow more aware of how your body feels, you will naturally connect to the subtle energies.

EXERCISE
Body to Soul Approach

Get settled into a chair in a space you find calm, safe, and sacred. As you are doing this, notice how your body feels. Pay attention to any thoughts that might be strumming in your mind. Be curious but not controlling of your state of being.

Now, imagine pulling in a blanket of safety around you. This is your sacred space, and no energy but yours can fill this room. Sit in this safe blanket and get adjusted to this energy for a while before you go on to the next part of the exercise.

Adjust the lighting, candles, diffusers, or whatever else helps you feel safe in the room. Grab your journal and a pen. You will close your eyes for this meditation, but keep these tools close by so you can do some channeled journaling.

Pull in several slow deep breaths from your nostrils and down to your belly. Take a minute to see yourself in the space. Notice the experience you are having as you sit and breathe.

Call attention to the pressure points in the seat. Wiggle your toes and move your feet around in a way that lets you experience being connected to the floor. Close your eyes and follow the breaths as you pull your attention inward.

- As you settle, bring your hand to your pelvic region and rest the palm over your pubic bone.
- Breathe into your hand. Connect with this portion of your body.
- This is the root chakra, the dimension of body and a connection to the earth.
- Allow yourself to deepen that connection by feeling yourself in the chair. Even move your toes a little more.
- Ask this area what it wants to tell you.

- Know that the answers may come as words in your head, memories, images, or other forms.
- Be open to the messages.
- As the information presents itself, draw or write the messages, keeping your eyes closed.
- Don't attempt to filter anything, as your reasoning brain will want to "make sense."
- When you feel the message are done, move your hand up to your abdomen. This is your sacral chakra, the home of early emotions and attachment.
- Feel the breath as your touch connects to this energy center. Take your time.
- Ask this energy what it wants to tell you.
- Stay open to anything that travels up to you.
- While keeping your eyes closed, take your pen and begin to draw or write the messages.
- When you feel all messages have finished, continue up to the solar plexus energy. This is the energy at the crux of your rib cage.
- See the connection of your hand as a welcoming partner with the energy.
- Breathe deep and expand your ribs. What does this information have to tell you? Take your time.
- When you feel you have all the information this area of your body is telling you in your journal, move your hand to the region of your heart.
- Breathe into your chest and pull the air deep into your lungs.

- Listen to what the heart chakra, the energy of compassion, has to say. Know that it holds truths that your mind does not understand.
- Draw, write, or scribble whatever it is telling you.
- When you are done, move your hand to your throat.
- Hold your hand gently along your throat chakra, the energy of compassion, and make sure your neck is extended but not tight.
- If this area of your body holds tension, let out a slow hum. There is no correct length of time for humming. Follow your intuition on this.
- Notice the sensation around your voice box as you do this.
- What information are you getting? Move your pencils on paper if there is more information your throat chakra wants to share.
- When you feel this information has completed itself, breathe into your throat. Thank it for what it had to say.
- Now settle the palm of your hand over your third eye, the energy of spirituality and your exclusive reality. Know that you have been using the energy all through this process as you attuned to the internal messages.
- Notice the sensation of holding your palm here.
- Create a soft smile on your face, as this loosens the many muscles in your face.
- Let these images fill the pages of your journal.
- When you feel the information has completed its cycle, move your hand to the top of your head.

- Take a second and settle your hand on the crown chakra, the energy of empathy and connection to the web of all life.
- Pause. Take your other hand and connect it back to your root chakra.
- Breathe into your belly and allow for a full circulation of energy from the crown to the root chakra. Spiritual to human experience.
- Settle into the energy for a time.
- Now, move your toes around.
- The energy of the crown and root chakras will engage in a cycle that continues to keep you grounded while you connect to a higher plane.
- Be with this experience.
- You can even keep one hand on your crown chakra and slide the other hand up along the sacral or solar plexus.
- What do you experience?

The last portion of this exercise was intended to help you see that you can stay in your body and still have that deep spiritual awareness. Too often people think being spiritual has a form of dissociation with it. The method here is to keep you connected to your body and listening to the messages it wants to share, not to have an out-of-body experience.

As you look back on this exercise, what are the patterns in your journal? They may not seem to make sense, or they could have a consistent message for you. When I do this sort of journaling, I find it might take weeks or months to understand the connected symbolism.

Notice the difference in how you feel now versus how you felt before this exercise. If you are feeling a need to write anything more in your journal, do so. Take this information that was given to you seriously. We are generally not taught to do bottom-up processing, so this keeps us suspicious of what we are taught. Were there health themes? Emotional themes? What did you glean?

Do this exercise anytime you feel the need to make a deep connection to all facets of you.

Seeking Solutions

The autonomic nervous system is the cornerstone of your health.[109] The vagus nerve releases a good portion of the hormones in your body to help the major organs function. Hormones that help keep emotional balance, such as oxytocin, epinephrine, and dopamine, come from the interplay of this nerve and your brain. Hormones that balance your sex drive are also innervated through the vagus nerve fibers.

A balanced system equates to better mood states—reason enough to continue to seek healthy solutions.

Supplementing the Vagus Nerve

When I discuss supplements, I am working from a place of my own writing (and some personal) research and not practicing medicine. Just as I stress to readers who are struggling with histories of high trauma to seek out a licensed trauma therapist, I strongly suggest you seek out a doctor of osteopathy or another licensed practitioner that can work systemically with you. These medical

---

109. Rosenberg, *Accessing the Healing Power of Your Vagus Nerve.*

professionals can run blood tests and personal diagnostics for you. If you are struggling with lethargy, anxiety, or depression, it's important to rule out larger issues.

How you feed your body affects your nervous system and brain.[110] In turn, all of this affects your way of being in the world. Let's start with some ways for you to supplement your nervous system.

Choline

Choline is vital for vagus nerve health.[111] This compound works similarly to vitamin B complex. Choline is the precursor to acetylcholine. Acetylcholine is the major neurotransmitter for the vagus nerve. Acetylcholine conducts information throughout the myelin sheaths of the nervous system. Choline is not classified as a vitamin or mineral. It has an amino acid–like makeup. In the last few decades, the focus on choline has increased.

The left hepatic branch of the vagus nerve connects to the liver. While your liver produces some choline, it is not enough for your nervous system to continue to repair itself, particularly if it's under a lot of stress. The research to determine the adequate amount of choline your body needs is not complete; however, a lack of choline can contribute to nonalcoholic forms of liver disease.

Any recommendations on proper amounts of choline for your body are going to be influenced by your medical practitioner and are exclusive to your needs.

Several decades ago, there used to be only food sources for choline. As research continues into how important this vitamin-like

---

110. Loper et al., "Both High Fat and High Carbohydrate Diets Impair Vagus Nerve Signaling of Satiety."
111. Kansakar, "Choline Supplements."

compound is for the sheaths of nerves, supplements have begun to appear on shelves. Choline can now be bought and taken in pill form.

The following is a list of some of the best food sources of choline.[112]

Liver: Both beef and chicken liver are some of the highest food sources for choline. For instance, beef liver has about 414 grams per ounce. Chicken liver has roughly 200 grams.

Eggs (yolks): Roughly 680 milligrams of choline are contained in 100 grams of egg yolk. Egg whites only contain 1 milligram per 100 grams. To get the nutritional benefits, eat the whole egg, particularly the egg yolk.

Beef: Some cuts of beef contain higher amounts of choline than others. Ground beef has upward of 100 milligrams per 1 cup. Other cuts, such as flank steak, have less.

Chicken breast: Chicken breast provides a high source of choline at 72 milligrams per 3-ounce serving.

Fish: Cold sea fish, such as Atlantic cod, have roughly 71 milligrams of choline per 3 ounces. This includes caviar, which has some of the highest amounts, and other fish roe, along with tuna and sardines.

Shitake mushrooms: Shitake mushrooms are packed with nutrients and have 27 milligrams of choline per ½ cup.

Cruciferous vegetables: Broccoli, cauliflower, brussels sprouts, and cabbage are good sources of choline.

---

112. Begum, "Top Foods High in Choline."

Soy: Tofu is higher in choline with 106 milligrams per 100 grams. Soy milk is lower with 56 milligrams. There are only trace amounts of choline in soybean oil.

Dairy: Milk, yogurt, and cheese are good sources of choline, though the amounts they have vary. For instance, 2 percent milk has roughly 40 milligrams of choline per 1 cup, while cheese has roughly 4.4 milligrams.

Other choline containing foods include red beans, red potatoes with skin, green peas, tangerines, carrots, apples, peanuts, brown rice, and sunflower seeds. Choline is water-soluble. That means you cannot store excess amounts in your system, as the mineral dissolves in water upon entering your body.

Magnesium

In my house, we jokingly refer to magnesium as the elixir of the gods.

Magnesium is one of the most common minerals on the earth. It plays a crucial role in managing sugar levels by modifying glucose and insulin. In women, magnesium helps to regulate many reproductive and gynecological issues, from premenstrual syndrome to menopause. This mineral is vital for good sleep, a sense of calm, better memory, and muscle and bone support. Magnesium activates adenosine triphosphate (ATP), which supports energy drive in the cells. Research shows magnesium is vital to maintaining brain neuroplasticity.[113]

It's important to know that magnesium plays a vital role in neuromuscular conduction, which is the electrical impulses sent

---

113. Li et al., "The Effect of Magnesium Alone or Its Combination with Other Supplements on the Markers of Inflammation, OS and Metabolism in Women with Polycystic Ovarian Syndrome (PCOS)."

through your nerves to help your muscles move. Magnesium transports calcium and potassium ions along the cell membranes. This contributes to regular nerve impulses and normal heart rhythm. Your autonomic nervous system needs healthy magnesium levels to function well. As we age, it's important to pay attention to magnesium levels, as they can decrease in older people who are on various medications.

Can't sleep? Try some magnesium supplements. While the research is mixed on why and if magnesium helps with sleep in certain populations,[114] many people try this mineral before bed. This is when I personally take mine, and I have found it to be vital to good rest. It is believed magnesium increases melatonin in the system.

Healthy amounts of magnesium can produce a natural sense of calm. Magnesium works on the benzodiazepine receptors in your brain in a natural way. These receptors are stimulated by and susceptible to Valium-type drugs, which are intended to induce calm. Benzodiazepine drugs can be very addictive.

Considering how well your body is holding and absorbing magnesium is vital. This mineral is processed through the gut, and the health of the gut plays a factor in more than 300 enzymatic reactions. As mentioned throughout this book, the gut-brain axis is key to a balanced autonomic nervous system. The recommended daily allowance for magnesium is 420 milligrams for adult males and 320 milligrams for adult females.[115]

About 50 to 60 percent of the total magnesium is stored in your bones. Another 40 to 50 percent is in your soft tissues and

---

114. Khalid, "Effects of Magnesium and Potassium Supplementation on Insomnia and Sleep Hormones in Patients with Diabetes Mellitus."
115. de Baaij et al., "Magnesium in Man."

muscles. Only about 2 percent is stored in red blood cells. Your kidneys, which are connected to your right (celiac) branches of your vagus nerve, manage the levels (homeostasis) of magnesium in your body.

Some foods high in magnesium are leafy green vegetables, edamame, kidney beans, pumpkin and chia seeds, almonds, peanuts, and cashews. Rice, both white and brown, and many cereal grains have magnesium. Chicken, fish, broccoli, carrots, and apples are decent sources as well.

There are several forms of magnesium, as it is bound with other minerals. The following is a generalized list of what they are and their functions.

> **Magnesium orotate:** One form of magnesium that speaks directly to our discussion on the vagus nerve is magnesium orotate. Orotate creates intercellular accumulation of magnesium, contributes to muscular endurance, and even has antitumor and antioxidant effects. This particular magnesium minimizes the damage of nerve cells and contributes to restoring cellular integrity of the nervous system tissues. The scientific community is exploring how magnesium orotate can alleviate neuropsychiatric disorders, as it relates to the brain-gut axis.[116]

> **Magnesium oxide:** Magnesium oxide is a form of magnesium salt that combines oxygen. It is used in antacids, as it helps with digestive issues. Because it doesn't absorb as well as other magnesium in the digestive tract, it is more frequently used to treat constipation or heartburn.

---

116. Schiopu et al., "Magnesium Orotate and the Microbiome-Gut-Brain Axis Modulation," 1567.

Magnesium citrate: This magnesium has a laxative effect, so use it accordingly. It is helpful for constipation but must be monitored as too much in the system can bring on diarrhea. This magnesium is bound to citric acid. Both magnesium oxide and magnesium citrate are not as effective in supporting brain health, but they are good for managing digestive issues.

Magnesium chloride: Magnesium chloride is utilized to treat type 2 diabetes, and there is much documentation about its efficacy. It is also used in treatment of high blood pressure, headaches, and osteoporosis.

Magnesium glycinate: Formed by combining magnesium with the amino acid glycine, this magnesium is rapidly absorbed in your lower intestines.

Magnesium malate: Magnesium malate combines magnesium and malic acid. It is believed to be a more rapidly absorbed form of the mineral. It can act as a laxative, so monitoring its effects is necessary.

Magnesium L-threonate: This magnesium has proven efficient at crossing the blood-brain barrier, which means it can impact brain health. Research is showing that magnesium L-threonate supports short- and long-term memory and may create new brain cells through stimulation of neurotransmitters.

Magnesium aspartate: Used to treat cardiac arrhythmias, magnesium aspartate is highly water soluble. It absorbs quickly into the bloodstream and is commonly used to treat magnesium deficiencies.

Magnesium malate: Stimulates ATP production and energizes the cells and muscular and nervous systems.

Magnesium taurate: Magnesium taurate is magnesium plus taurine, which is an amino acid. Taurine works as a neurotransmitter in the brain and has been used to treat hyperactivity, high blood pressure, and heart rate issues.

EXERCISE
Recipe: Treating Your Nervous System and Chakras to a Magnesium Soak

Out of desperation one day, I meditated and came up with this exercise. At one of the hardest times during an illness I had with shingles (more on that later), I could not get my inflammation down. At the risk of overselling this experience, and also making it clear this was experimental for myself and doesn't carry scientific validity, I want to share that the day following it, I woke up with no inflammation. After a brief stomach upset, things cleared out of my system. I felt completely better. From that day forward, I was on the upswing with my health, as long as I watched the things for me that create inflammation and stayed on my medicine.

I can't make those promises for you. We are all different, and I am not a medical doctor. Certainly, magnesium salt baths are a common recommendation by many practitioners. If you feel confident enough to try this, know that, at the very least, this technique can't hurt.

There is some preparation involved, which is why I'm calling this exercise a recipe.

What you will be doing is making magnesium packets by putting the salts in 6 × 6–inch squares of cheese cloth. Then you will incorporate some castor oil (organic and in a glass jar) over bare skin on each energy center. You will then rest the packets on five of the seven chakra centers, using warm water in a spray bottle to wet the packets. Expect to get a good rest as you let them sit there and soak for thirty to sixty minutes (depending on your patience). It's also a bit messy, so you will needs lot of towels to lay on.

Here's my theory about why treatment worked so well.

As described earlier, each of the chakras is an extension of the vagus nerve endings or nerve plexuses. As the castor oil and magnesium soak into the energy centers, they reach deep into the nervous system. Your major digestive organs are getting a healthy dose of anti-inflammation components from the magnesium. The castor oil is also an anti-inflammatory product and has been known to cleanse the liver and digestive system as it soaks into your skin.[117] Given how soothing magnesium is for the body, you can do this before bed. It gave me a good night's sleep.

You will need to be unclothed for this exercise, as things get a bit drippy.

Materials
- Cheesecloth
- Scissors
- 24 inches of thin twine cut into five 4-inch-long pieces
- 1 jar magnesium chloride flakes. I have a large jar of flakes that I also use as bath salts.
- Organic castor oil (stored in a glass bottle). These are usually sold in 8-ounce sizes.
- Two to three large, thick bathroom towels
- Small spray bottle filled with filtered, warm water

---

117. Vieira et al., "Effect of Ricinoleic Acid in Acute and Subchronic Experimental Models of Inflammation."

Preparation

- Make five 6 × 6–inch square cuts of cheesecloth. The cheesecloth comes folded once. Keep it folded, as the double layer provides enough hold yet enough porousness to allow the minerals to seep through.
- On the middle of each square, put 1 tablespoon of magnesium flakes.
- Pull the sides of the cloth together and twist it closed.
- Use twine to tie the cloth closed, making a small pouch.
- The twine usually sticks well enough that one tie will hold. If not, double knot it.
- Lay down several towels, making sure they will extend from the top of your head down to your knees. Make sure the towels are wide enough to catch any magnesium that may drip off you.
- Rub a sufficient amount of castor oil on your root, sacral, solar plexus, heart, and throat chakras. I would say about a teaspoon. If you are inclined, you can run the oil along the whole length of your torso or the nadis that connect to the chakras.
- Wet each magnesium pouch by spraying with the warm water. Then rest one pouch on each chakra.
- If you are chilly, you can put a towel over you.
- Simply enjoy the rest for thirty to sixty minutes. (Don't fall asleep yet.)
- When you are done, you can remove the balls and toss them out.
- Take a warm shower after you are done since your skin will feel "salty."

- Notice how your system responds over the next several hours. Or enjoy your sleep.

If you like, you can find a nice crystal point to rest at the top of your head near the crown chakra, but this doesn't impede the effects of this process.

Enjoy.

Food Matters

Food, in its simplest description, is energy. A "Westernized" diet that is composed of too much processed food depletes your system. Many other related behaviors do, too, such as the use of diuretics, which reduces minerals and vitamins that your body needs. Certainly, eating disorders and disordered eating, including restriction and binge-purging, destroy your body's natural balance.[118] This affects not only your physical well-being but your mental health because these behaviors are exhausting your nervous system and vagal tone.

Many minerals are necessary to maintain proper functioning of your nervous system. These include calcium, potassium, selenium, zinc, sodium, iron, copper, manganese, and iodine. They contribute to electrolyte balance. Proper electrolyte balance is also important to the health of your cerebrospinal fluid, that colorless liquid that surrounds the brain and spinal cords and helps conduct signals throughout your whole body.

Making sure your body does not suffer from vitamin deficiencies is also important. B group vitamins (such as B12, B6, B4, and B1) and vitamin C are water-soluble, which means they don't have

---

118. Melis et al., "Trans-Auricular Vagus Nerve Stimulation in the Treatment of Recovered Patients Affected by Eating and Feeding Disorders and Their Comorbidities."

a dangerous buildup in your system. Vitamins D and E, which are not water-soluble, along with vitamin C help manage inflammation in your body.[119] Inflammation is the cause of so many health-related problems.

The presence of antioxidants in the diet protects against oxidative damage to nervous system cells. Biochemical data indicate that polyunsaturated fatty acids such as arachidonic acid (AA), docosahexaenoic acid (DHA), cicosatetraenoic acid (EPA), and gamma-linolenic acid (GLA) play a key role in contributing to nervous system function.[120] Tryptophan, phenylalanine, tyrosine, taurine, glucose, and beta-carotene are also important. They can be absorbed in your body through foods.

Beta-Blockers

Beta-blockers are drugs used to manage heart rhythm and reduce high blood pressure. Some doctors use beta-blockers with patients who have experienced high levels of stress or trauma to reduce levels of stress in the body.[121]

These medicines work by blocking the hormone adrenaline (or epinephrin). The heart beats more slowly and with less intensity as the veins and arteries widen. This improves blood flow. Beta-blockers reduce sympathetic activity and may increase parasympathetic (ventral vagal) activity. Before even considering this as an option for stress management, you must consult with your medical doctor.

---

119. Shaik-Dasthagirisaheb et al. "Role of Vitamins D, E and C in Immunity and Inflammation," 291–95.
120. Harwood, "Polyunsaturated Fatty Acids."
121. Van der Kolk, *The Body Keeps the Score*, 123.

Other Medical Treatments to Manage Nerve Health

Antiviral medicines have been able to curb viral loads from the nerve fibers that are "loaded" into the blood and affect the rest of the body. A viral load is the number of viral particles found in the blood. Some viruses, such as the human immunodeficiency virus (HIV), herpes simplexes (HSV), and varicella-zoster virus (VZY), hide in the nervous system and reappear during times of stress.

Cindy's Story: Deciding to Stay

My client Cindy was a retired pediatrician that I had seen years earlier due to childhood trauma. She returned because she had just experienced the loss of three close family members, including her adult child. With so many impacts to her nervous system, she was not only emotionally struggling, but her immune system was starting to shut down. She struggled with sleeping and eating. She became severely immunocompromised and depressed.

Cindy was determined to find hope and move beyond these losses. She said she felt they were opportunities to grow spiritually. Besides, she said, she really didn't have much choice but to try to find hope again.

Her resolve deeply moved me. None of us know how we would act in such situations until we are faced with them. I was in awe of how deeply within herself she was reaching. The best I could do as her therapist was companion her through this sometimes-brutal journey.

The years progressed and Cindy found meaning and some relief.

"Time does soften the blow," she said. "The losses, especially of my child, don't seem so on top of me but rolling alongside of me now."

Despite her determination to heal, Cindy continued to struggle with health issues. Her energy was drained, and she said she was not able to breathe deeply. She could not cross the street without having to sit down to rest.

Cindy said her heart rate was fine. Given her own medical background and despite extensive testing, she could not find a medical reason for this. The best she could discern was that her lungs were not connecting with her autonomic nervous system.

"I've looked at all the research; there is no medical framework or protocol for this problem," she said. "I have been to my cardiologist, pulmonologist, and even a neurologist. Every test comes back fine."

"Well," I said, "maybe it's time to listen to your intuition. It has been serving you well as you have managed your grief."

To manage her sleepless nights, Cindy had taken to meditation several hours a day. She said she found it helpful. Cindy left that session stating she would meditate on her physical issues and see what appeared.

"I have nothing to lose," she said.

She came back the next week looking a little better but still very tired. "Magnesium and potassium," she said.

"What do you mean?"

"That's what kept coming to me during meditation."

"And?"

"I've started on regular doses. I'm adding other electrolytes, and I'm feeling a little better."

It wasn't up to me to argue one way or another with a medical doctor who had combed through all the research. "Well, it's certainly not going to hurt. You know more than anyone the correct dosages."

Cindy said she believed that her body had gone through such a shock that it wanted to stop all life functions. "The trauma has been so hard on my system," she said. "However, I believe my Soul wants to stay."

"That is profound," I said.

"I still have work to do down here." She was quiet for a while. "Copper, magnesium, potassium, and zinc," she said. "That's random but not really." After a few more seconds she said, "It's all the minerals the nervous system needs anyway. I both know this and got a gut check about it."

"Excellent!"

"It's also these minerals that the Soul needs to continue to interact with our body," she said. "We can die if we are depleted of these minerals, and we die because the Soul cannot connect to the system."

"Wow," I said. This woman was a constant amazement to me.

"You're right." She laughed. "Our vagus nerve is the Soul nerve."

She talked about breath techniques as well.

"My Soul wants back in," she said.

Through the next few months, Cindy's energy increased. She worked with a shamanic healer along the way, and she stated they helped her to understand herself and what she had already seen regarding what she saw as the separation of her Soul from the body.

"It would leave so often, especially at night, that my body struggled to integrate with it at times."

"Something tells me that one's not going into the medical journals," I said.

She shrugged. "Who knows. Maybe so. I'm thinking of starting an alternative medicine practice. Nothing like having a left and right brain approach to healing."

Cindy's face appeared brighter and happier as time went on. She moved more freely, and her breathing skills increased. Her eyes had more sparkle, and she was more animated.

"I went for a run the other day," she said. "I haven't done that in years."

"Fantastic!"

"I'll see them again one day," Cindy said. "I know they are there with me, watching over me. They will help me as I start this next leg of my journey."

Summary

Over the last few decades, it's become deeply understood that the autonomic nervous system is the major foundation of all that is important in physical wellness and optimal emotional functioning. The vagus nerve releases a good portion of the hormones in your body to help the major organs work efficiently. Hormones that help keep emotional balance, such as oxytocin, epinephrine, and dopamine, come from the interplay of this nerve and your brain. Hormones that balance your sex drive are also interplayed through the innervation of the vagus nerve fibers. A balanced system means more balanced hormones, which equates to better mood states. Food, especially those containing choline, are optimal for vagus nerve health, as choline is a precursor to the major neurotransmitter of acetylcholine, which makes up your myelinated sheaths. Electrolytes, minerals, and vitamins are also vital contributors to your vagal and overall health.

PART 3
THE JOURNEY ON YOUR TERMS

CHAPTER 8
YOUR INTERNAL NATURE HEALS

•——————•

This is the chapter where I get a bit personal. Due to various stressors, I got a nice bout of shingles during the time I was writing this book. Ironically, I was researching the chapter on vagus nerve health. My doctor and I had a good laugh over that.

Shingles is a viral infection caused by the same virus responsible for chicken pox. After you recover from chicken pox, the virus lies dormant in your body's nerve tissue near the spinal cord and brain. Decades later, that virus can flare up because of stressors and age. Once it's reactivated, the shingles virus travels along nerve fibers to the skin. This causes a painful rash. Shingles appears as a band on one side of the body. That pattern corresponds to the affected nerves.

"Perhaps," my doctor said, "you are being given some great insights to write about."

She wasn't kidding. However, as we've all experienced at times, some of the best lessons are not the easiest ones. It was the depths of winter and despite religiously taking my prescribed meds, the virus would not tamp down. So, I went deep into meditation. Just like with Cindy's story, there is great wisdom when you access your inner world to ask for healing guidance. The information that comes out of those meditation sessions might not make sense at first. The key is to trust enough to get it written or drawn. You can then revisit that information later.

How I did this for myself was to settle into my chair and place a notepad and pen beside me. I used many of the breathing techniques I've led you through in this book. When I felt centered enough, I asked to be shown what I could do to heal my nervous system more rapidly. Eventually, information came though images and sometimes words I heard in my head. As I listened, I wrote. This is the tricky part since the brain wants to jump in with its prescribed knowledge. Without analyzing the information, I just kept writing and drawing. Some very interesting exercises came about.

Always the clinician that likes to verify, after I received this information, I went immediately into research mode. With these exercises I am sharing in this chapter, I am able to tell you why they work from a neurobiological as well as an energetic standpoint. I'm also able to tell you from personal experience that they made a huge difference in my recovery.

Every person and every body is different. I cannot substantiate how well these exercises will help you. They have only been tested on me. If none of them feel right to you, please don't pursue them.

I would also encourage you to do your own meditation "asks" regarding your health. Further into the chapter I will break that process down for you. Your Soul wisdom cannot lead you astray once you are able to connect and communicate with it.

Here are the exercises I was shown. I'm very excited to share these with you! I'm also excited to let you know that I'm doing great now. While it was a rough road for a bit, I believe following my internal wisdom sped up my healing. Trust your wisdom. Soul has a natural inclination toward healing—so does your body. Soul will always rise to a higher frequency to help your human parts along.

Fields, Streams, and Mountains

The first section of exercises is a series of breathing meditations. There are a few steps to these, so I have given you diagrams to help you envision them. If you have been working through the previous breathing techniques, you will find these to be very doable.

These exercises spoke directly to what I have learned over the years about the vagus nerve and chakra energy. So, I understood why I was being directed to do them. I then found more clinical evidence through modalities such as Feldenkrais techniques and other physical therapy modalities to back up the "whys." This breath work and movement of the diaphragmatic and subdiaphragmatic branches of the vagus nerve is a nice reset that balances out your system.

Let's go through them. Know that you don't need shingles or any other inflammatory issues to benefit from them. These exercises will bring you relief if you are struggling with stressors or relaxing, and I would highly suggest you integrate them into the maintenance of your overall well-being, as intentional breath can do.

EXERCISE
Mountain then Valley

I call this exercise series Mountain then Valley, as it has a rolling rhythm that conjures up the green mountains of Wales for me. With every mountain, there is a valley below it. This healing journey through life seems to have a similar undulating pattern. As a result, Mountain then Valley awakens the healing nature that is already within you. I believe it has also helped to engage my vagus nerve in a way that actively took down a lot of my inflammation, as breath can do. As I said, done lovingly, at the very least this exercise is not going to hurt you.

Mountain Breathing

This first step in Mountain then Valley is called Mountain Breathing. It is a deep chest breath. It expands your lungs, involves your pectoralis major muscle and upper ribs, and opens up the heart chakra as it brings energy to your lungs and heart. This engages the ventral vagal complex of the vagus nerve.

The intake and outbreath breaths have to be done slowly, just like you have learned. Be patient and kind to yourself as you do this breathing exercise. The setup looks like this:

- This exercise is done with you lying down on your back, but if you struggle with this, you most certainly can sit.
- You can either rest on the floor, a yoga mat, or a bed. Your position needs to be secure.
- If you are lying, make sure your legs are slightly elevated with a pillow or other bolster under your knees. This flattens your lower back and keeps your feet firmly planted.
- You will also need a small pillow to support your head without bending your neck too far backward or forward. The objective is to keep your airways open.
- Rest your arms alongside your body with palms up.
- Palms facing up squares your shoulders but also softens them into a position where they won't roll forward as you breathe deeply.

- With lips closed, let your jaw relax, as if you are asleep.
- If you are familiar with yoga practices, this resting position looks like a very supported savasana (dead man's pose).

Here we go:

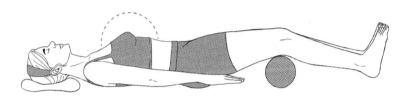

Figure 8: Mountain Breathing

- Relax your whole face.
- Imagine the muscles from your hairline and along your brow, eyes, and cheeks melting into the ground.
- *Slowly* take in a deep, long breath through the nostrils.
- Pull the breath all the way down into the lungs.
- Let the chest expand as you fill your lungs.
- This should almost feel unnatural, as we don't usually breathe this generously into our chest.
- Imagine the air spreading out to fill the chest cavity.
- Hold.
- *Slowly* exhale through the nose.
- Wait a beat, then do it again.
- Notice the breath as it comes in through the nostrils, down the back of the throat, and deep into the bottom of the lungs.
- Feel this expansion along your upper spine.

- Hold again, then observe as the air releases from the lungs, travels along the throat, and makes its way back out the nasal passages.
- Do this about ten times.
- Stretch then slowly sit up.
- Explore how your body feels.
- Are you still breathing deeply? Has anything changed for you?

Expanding your upper ribs with breath brings room to your thoracic and cervical spine. Your breath is working your system more deeply. This massages the organs of the heart, lungs, and upper digestive tract to balance your heart rate. As you do this, be curious about the energy in your neck, throat, jaw, and ears. This area of your body is a relay center for your sensory nerves. As you continue to breathe in deeper ways, your whole system will register this as more normal and it will become natural.

Eventually, you will alternate phase one (Mountain Breathing) and phase two (Valley Breathing), but for now, let's get a feel for each step. Are you ready for step 2? We will practice this on its own, then eventually incorporate them.

Valley Breathing

This phase is called Valley Breathing, which is diaphragmatic. Your stomach will move up and down like the undulations of a valley. Diaphragmatic breathing is what you have been doing throughout book.

You will start in the same supine position that you did with step 1 of this exercise. Relax your body, facial muscles, and tongue. Keeping lips closed, get used to breathing through your nose for a second. Again, make sure your head is supported in a position that allows the air to flow. This time you will be pulling deep, slow breaths down into your lower abdomen, expanding the muscles until they create a nice round belly for you. Here we go:

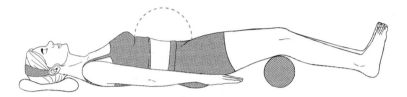

Figure 9: Valley Breathing

- Pull in a breath through your nostrils and drag the air down into your lower belly.
- Imagine the light of your root chakra expanding as you do this.
- Let the belly expand and soften.
- Don't worry as much about expanding the ribs. Focus on letting the abdominal muscles soften and expand.
- Hold for as long as you can.
- *Slowly* release the breath.
- Use your abdominal muscles to expel the air.
- Keep your face, tongue, and throat soft as you do this.
- Do this sequence again and imagine the air moving into your root chakra.
- Slowly breathe out.
- Breathe into the sacral chakra.
- Exhale.
- Breathe into the solar plexus chakra.
- Exhale.
- Continue this cycle for as long as you would like.

It takes some time to break the habit of chest-only breath-ing. If you have been studying yoga for a while, abdominal or diaphragmatic breathing is one of the techniques you regularly practice. However, you don't have to take weekly yoga classes to learn this way of drawing air into your belly. Just put intention toward the experience. Over time, it will come as your muscles relearn.

Take a moment, sit up, and check in with your body. What do you notice. This diaphragmatic breathing is soothing the sympathetic branch of the vagus along and engaging the dor-sal vagal branch, which is bringing life into the visceral organs. This at once calms and energizes you.

Don't jump into step 3 of this exercise right away. Take a few days to practice step 1 (Mountain Breathing) and step 2 (Valley Breathing). Only when you are ready, do both together, as this creates a rolling or alternating experience in your system and takes some work and pacing.

Rolling from Mountain to Valley

Now, let's bring in the undulating Mountain then Valley as we combine these two breathing movements. The combination is not to do both chest and belly expansion at the same time. The intention with this third step in the exercise is to expand, then release the chest (Mountain), then expand and release the belly (Valley). It seems to create a pleasant kneading motion between the upper and lower diaphragmatic portions of your vagus nerve.

I can't stress enough for you to do these intakes and out-breaths slowly. You are expanding your system in ways you may not have before; breathing too rapidly might create hyperventi-lation, so be mindful of the experience.

Let's start with the upper torso breathing, then alternate to the lower section, then back up again.

Here we go:

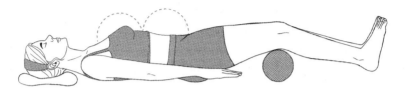

Figure 10: Mountain then Valley

- While lying in a supine position, notice if your muscles have tensed at all. If so, go through a body scan of softening the face, tongue, and throat. Let the jaw slack while keeping lips closed.
- Pull your breath into the lower portion of your lungs and hold for five seconds (Mountain).
- Slowly release as you follow the sensation of the exhale.
- Wait for two counts, then breathe into your belly (Valley) and hold.
- Release slowly.
- Wait for two counts, then breathe deep into the lungs (Mountain) and hold.
- Alternate this upper breath, then lower breath several times.

Perform as many repetitions as you can, then just lie still for a while. Be present and notice how you feel. This process forces you to be intentional. It increases the awareness of your body and breath. If you notice tense muscles, release them. The only system that should be doing any work is your respiratory system. The respiratory system in this case is not only the respiratory diaphragm but the pelvic and the laryngeal diaphragms (pelvis and throat).

Why This Deeply Changes Things

Valley then Mountain is a great soother and activator of the whole vagus nerve, all the organs and, of course, the chakras. It's pulling air into your system in ways you probably haven't done before.

The first step engages the safety branch of the vagus nerve, which is ventral vagal activation. A deep breath in activates; a slow exhale calms. It makes room for the heart and lungs and lowers blood pressure.

You will naturally experience the energy shifts in the heart, throat (which includes middle ear), and third eye chakras. This breathing also settles the brain into a sense of calm and engages the higher reasoning functions in the prefrontal lobe. Mountain Breathing takes your brain out of a reactionary mode because you are sending signals of safety to your system.

The second phase of this exercise, Valley Breathing, engages sympathetic and dorsal branches to collaborate in safety. Both are engaged but not over- or underactivated. The air being pulled into your tummy works almost like a massage to the deeper organs. This is the rest and digest branch in your body.

According to several physical therapy methods, loosening the jaw in this way naturally brings pelvic alignment.[122] Of course, with an aligned pelvis and skull, you experience an easy flow of nervous system and chakra energy.

---

122. Feldenkrais, *The Elusive Obvious.*

Tapping Your Highest Potential

Every healing modality that has come into the world was given to its architect from a higher Source. From medicines that cured deadly diseases and meditation or energy styles of healing to psychological theories and methods, they were all streaming out there on various universal wave lengths that people tapped into. Whether they knew it or not, these scientists were vibing with the cosmos before they worked out models with their intellect.

We are not so powerful alone. Our power comes when we can open to the infinite wisdom that is wanting to work through us. Being able to understand we are the channelers of that information, not the ultimate creators of it, takes enough humility to form that information into a clear foundation for others.

That doesn't mean we are powerless. We have free will. Within that will we need to cultivate our education and skill sets so we can do the work and relay that information well. Learning new technological platforms, communicating efficiently, or deeply studying an ancient modality develops a foundation that we can springboard from.

To be open to that flow of information requires that you engage with your body—in safety. You can't access a deeper flow if your neurobiology thinks it has to be on high alert because it feels little more than fear. While the openness of the crown and third eye chakras engages in being aware of higher frequencies and information, your essential chakras are keeping you grounded to accept this information. This is why it's important that your nervous system works in an effective manner. It's got to succinctly interpret information that comes your way.

How to tap in with the highest intention is where you thrive. When you are content being still, you can access your internal world. That Soul is a lodestone for the higher information that is wanting to tell you something. Feeling safe in your body lets you make room in your busy head and aching heart to listen closer.

Part of this is trusting the training you have chosen so you can effectively design, implement, or discover the next healing mode for humanity. An example of having competencies in place to bring in a new way to heal is Francine Shapiro, the developer of EMDR. Her personal experience around REM led her to explore using eye movements with her traumatized clients. Over time, with academic research, she advanced studies around how effective this was. A brand-new understanding that shifted the way therapists help heal trauma was born. From EMDR has come other neurobiological modalities, such as Brainspotting. It was Shapiro's education and experience that helped her launch EMDR into the world in a way she would not have been able to if she wasn't already a trauma-informed psychologist. Yet, it was her tapping into a frequency of healing for herself that inspired EMDR.[123]

We pass up amazing ideas and opportunities all the time. Sometimes, it's because we're worried someone or the great-judgmental-something-or-other is going to negate them. Fear of failing or fear of being so successful we might rise beyond where we are keeps us from being true to ourselves.

The phrase *fear of the unknown* is really not an unknown. That is because your mind has already projected fear into the future. Your mind already believes it will know what will happen. What it fears will happen has been defined by your thoughts based on old messages and past experiences. Fear will haunt you if you let it. So, understand that the important thing about fear is it's in your

---

123. Shapiro, *Getting Past Your Past*.

imagination. You can move beyond it. Keep walking. You'll get past that imaginary space soon enough.

As one dear writer friend joked to me decades ago while he was writing a book about his time in Vietnam, "Showing your ass in public is scarier than fighting a war, sometimes. At least in war you've been trained. You never know what the critics are going to say about your art."

Author and researcher Brene Brown has certainly helped us all to normalize those fears of doing something authentic in front of others.[124] Be scared, worried, uncertain, fearful, and nervous, and do it anyway. Your mind will seek out fears and send faulty neuroception to your system. You know this now.

Because you are becoming aware of this "fear of the unknown," you can learn to manage it better while you're in the midst of it. It's sometimes pushing through on that hillside walk that gets you to the top—not in total ease but through the discomfort of knowing there is a higher, wiser intention at play and knowing you are actually safe.

Reaching your Soul through the fear is where you tap into the creative forces that uniquely blend with your talents. Your talents, particular your style and drive to know, is your Soul. We don't want to pull back from this. Trust that your Soul knows more than your ego parts do and listen. Be patient.

Remember that leading a spiritual path does not take you out of the world but keeps you engaged more fully in it. That includes understanding what contributions you can bring to it. Fear of success or failure has some deep, dark channels, but it is never more powerful than your eternal light.

---

124. Brown, *I Thought It Was Just Me.*

The following is an example of one person who had all the ideas streaming in his head but was terrified to implement them.

Blake's Story: Fear of the Unknown

Blake was twenty-five years old when he came to see me. A brilliant visual artist and musician, he stated his anxiety was too high for him to perform with his band anymore.

He said there was a lot of conflict in the group because they needed him to keep things together and he couldn't. Blake's heritage was Puerto Rican, Swedish, and African American. He spent his childhood in Europe, throughout the Caribbean, and in the States. He joked that his cultural influences all competed against each other.

His Swedish mother was a doctor. She would take him and his sister on mission trips across the globe as she worked with Doctors Without Borders. His father was a painter, and while he loved to travel, he complained that following his wife around the world kept him from having any success of his own.

Blake said his parents were separated and had been since he was a teen. His sister was in New York City in medical school, and he hadn't seen her in a year.

"Dad still hasn't had any success," Blake said, "even though he's been in one place, his hometown, for ten years now. Mostly he sips liquor and contemplates what he will put on the canvas."

"He sounds a little stalled himself," I said.

There was a moment of silence as Blake stared at me. "Oh wow, yeah. You're right."

Blake played saxophone and guitar. His genre was a form of jazz fusion. He showed me some videos. They were spectacular.

As his band performed on stage, they would project Blake's mixed-media artwork behind them. Through some amazing technical artistries that were beyond my knowledge, his art moved and responded to his notes. Blake's creations were compelling and engaged all the senses. To my untrained ear, his music was polished. His visual art manipulated color and form and kept you mesmerized.

"Wow," I said. "This is professional. Looks like you're on the brink of something big."

"Yeah," he said. His voice faded.

The man sitting in front of me did not represent the energy he projected on stage. He was underweight, pale, not sleeping, and fearful. His uncertain presence seemed incongruent to that larger-than-life performance I just saw on his social media feed.

I smiled and leaned forward. Blake's wide eyes showed sadness as he looked back at me.

"What part scares you the most?" I asked.

He was silent a while. I waited.

Then he said, "Being seen." He shook his head. "Scares the shit out of me."

"I understand," I said. "Sometimes, it's easier to stay in the background."

The more we talked, the more I could hear the echoes of trauma in his family's history. Despite his continental, expansive upbringing, he seemed reluctant to live a bigger life. Yet, he also seemed driven to do so.

There was nothing overt—no beatings, shouting, molestations, or verbal abuse—in Blake's childhood. Both Blake's mother and father had experienced these things and swore they would never do this to their children. However, unresolved trauma trickles down in psychic waves if it is not healed. It can be experienced covertly.

While there was no shouting in Blake's household, both parents, when they could no longer connect because of their childhood wounds, retreated in icy silence. Silent resentment became the foundation of Blake's family connection. Staying angry, with no words, was the painful bond that Blake and his sister watched and learned from.

Eventually, his mother threw herself into healing "the world," as Blake put it, and his father continued to complain that Blake's mother was the cause of his inability to create. Over the years, as the oldest sibling, Blake started to feel his role was the peacemaker between his parents. He watched his mother's world expand with work and travel while silently covering up her own unhappiness. He felt compelled to encourage his father with his creativity, but that effort bore no fruit. Both parents used Blake as the sounding board for their own misery.

"How do you feel now?" I asked. "Do you still feel torn between your parents?"

"Yes," he said, "but I don't want to be."

"Let's not worry about outcome," I said. "Let's worry about healing process. Whatever comes out of this, artistically or otherwise, is the way it's supposed to be."

"Cool," he said. "How do we do that?"

We started by exploring family messaging that came down from as many generations as Blake knew of. We explored his own beliefs based on this versus what felt true to him. He needed the time and space to even know what his truth was. Blake came to understand that we cannot heal ourselves by trying to fix others. Attempting to fix others was just a preoccupation from healing himself.

"So," he joked one day, "if I'm working on me, I can't blame them, can I?"

"Yeah, you know," I joked back, "that taking responsibility for ourselves thing is the ultimate adulting, isn't it?"

Over time, Blake said his playing got easier and the conflict in his band lessened. His creativity was taking all sorts of interesting turns. Blake realized his thinking was backward. He thought angst was at the core of all creativity.

"That starving, tortured artist thing," he said. "I think I was afraid to get rid of it. That I wouldn't have anything to express if I did."

"Angst," I said, "is just another attempt at controlling things we can't control."

"I see that in my dad." Blake looked over at me. "I don't want to be like him."

"Instead of worrying if you are or aren't like him, just know yourself deeply," I said. "That way, you can work from your own core and not spend your life pushing back against his choices."

"Identifying with being sick doesn't keep you safe, does it?" he asked.

"Nope," I said. "It just keeps you sick."

EXERCISE
Releasing the Dam

This exercise engages the throat while gently innervating the auricular nerve in the vagus. The auricular provides sensory innervation to the outside of the auditory canal and the outer surface of the eardrum. Stimulating the auricular might trigger a cough, which is called Arnold's reflex.

You will be gently inserting your finger halfway into your ear, so please use caution. If you have long nails, you will need to modify this exercise by lightly rubbing the outside of the ear fold. You will also be humming a soft, long frequency. Use the chant of "ohmmm" since this extends the vibration. Yogis have known for centuries that your fingers possess their own chakric flow of energy. Studies indicate that the pointer finger expends the strongest of some of that energy.[125]

Do this exercise slowly. If you feel uncomfortable at all (which goes for any exercises), do not proceed.

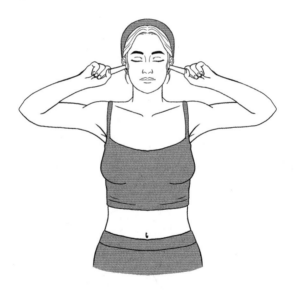

Figure 11: Releasing the Dam

---

125. Jabs and Rubik, "Detecting Subtle Energies with a Physical Sensor Array."

- Lift your arms out, then point your fingers toward your ears, keeping your elbows extended while you slip your index fingers in your ears.
- Your elbows remain extended out in order to open the chest and give room for the ventral vagal complex.
- Apply a reasonable amount of pressure into the ears. Use reason and caution as to how far you go.
- Close your eyes.
- Soften your jaw and keep your lips together.
- Allow your facial muscles to "melt" like they did in the previous exercises.
- Take a deep into your lungs.
- Hold breath for five seconds.
- With eyes closed, hum a long, slow "ohmmm" chant.
- Continue this process for as long as you want.

Healing Is the Journey

There seems to be an unspoken assumption with any healing process, including trauma work, that there is a perfect state of being attained at the end of treatment. Worse, there also seems to be an unspoken belief that if you aren't flawlessly healed, *you* are the problem. Not true. Healing, growth, understanding—it is as a lifelong process. There is not an "end goal" where we find ourselves free of burdens and with perfect insight. Each layer of healing brings on a deeper awareness and ability to reach another pathway.

What the Soul does not ask for is avoidance of the path, regardless of what your journey looks like. The body, in its programming to keep you safe, develops strategies to avoid danger. Our wiring, through our brain and nervous system, stores information that makes us act from fear, which might look like avoidance. That, however, is a wonderful sign to ask for guidance.

Summary

Be open to the flow within you. When you are able to sit quietly and listen, information that can guide you will become available. It is natural to doubt that information, but give it time and just sit with it. Your body has an incredible ability to heal itself if you allow the space for the healing. When you heal physically, you alleviate emotional blockages that stifle creativity and interpersonal experiences. Creating that safe space around you is important. Listen, be still, and be honest with what is right for you. You can't access a deeper flow if your neurobiology thinks it has to be on high alert. Take the time to calm your body. Be patient with yourself.

CHAPTER 9
REACHING YOUR SOUL
BY WAY OF VAGAL TONE

What happens when you're not afraid? How do you experience that in your body? What happens when you become afraid? Are you able to bring yourself back to a centered presence when all indications are that you're safe? How well you can reclaim a feeling of steadiness after an upsetting event or stressful encounter is an indicator of your vagal tone.

Vagal tone is everything we have covered in this book so far. It is a measure of the influence of the vagus nerve on your heart and respiratory functioning. High vagal tone means you have good physical and emotional health. It indicates a strong heart, a strong gut microbiome, and a strong immune system. Low vagal tone, on the other hand, is linked to high levels of chronic stress, which brings on inflammation and many health conditions that we covered in previous chapters.

How well you can slow down your heart rate and promote a state of calm and relaxation is the best indicator of vagal health. You can increase vagal tone by making changes in your overall lifestyle. This is the way in.

What You Get by Calming Your System

What do you get by calming your system? Peace. Spiritual and psychological maturity. Inner knowing. Self-love that extends more easily and in healthy ways to others. Oh, and access to the greatest knowledge you can possess, which, of course, comes from your Soul. Your inner compass is handed back to you.

Having an ability to bounce back in situations because you can reclaim safety in your nervous system settles you on to your very right and true pathway. You understand which way to go. You possess ownership of your life with a power to decide.

As we discussed in previous chapters, working from the premise that your Soul chose this life changes everything. Coming here was part of a greater plan that your Soul energy requested. You were not randomly tossed into the world and its uncertainty without a plan, purpose, and map forward.

Creating life through your Soul also helps you to know you are never alone. This way of being is the major theme as you work through this book. Shift your patterns within yourself now, and you can create forward motion in your life. Sometimes, this shift takes more work than other times, but the outcome leads to peace.

Allowing your Soul to lead the way is like utilizing and trusting your factory-installed inner compass. It guides you through the good times as well as the awful ones. You need to rely on it.

Past-life regressionists have asked "how" for decades. Their work continues to shake up the stagnant thinking about life direction and pushes us beyond the basic scope of the mind.

According to the Michael Newton Institute of Life Between Lives, your Soul chose where and with whom you are living on this planet.[126] Dolores Cannon and Brian Weiss, also pioneers with greater questions, indicated through their hypnotherapy sessions with thousands of clients that the Soul seeks a completion of understanding on this earth. They have learned the Soul cannot be destroyed, unlike the body. They confirmed simple knowledge—that people tend to complicate—that once Soul leaves, the body decays. They have also learned that your Soul wants wonderful things for you.[127] So, let's make the best of this by honoring its choices.

Grace and genuineness are Soul energy. Let us do the human work of continuing to access it while we are here. Let us take the time and space to understand what we need know. That is true strength. Your life is a psychologically spiritual process.

Hello, Old Friend

You have met your Soul, even if the moments appear fleeting. Like a familiar friend, it has been there waiting for you to notice it again.

Your Soul possesses a wisdom that your brain and body—despite their amazing messaging systems—cannot know. From the simplest of truths about the next thing you need to do in your life to the more complex understanding of where you came from, your Soul holds an infinite database of knowledge that extends beyond your limited human experience.

You can't think of Soul and have it appear since it's always there.

While Soul is not of the mind, Soul is very aware of your mind's existence. Mind, however, is not so aware of the Soul. Conceptually, mind knows something is there. However, the work of

---

126. Newton, *Journey of Souls*.
127. Cannon, *Between Death and Life*; Weiss, *Many Lives, Many Masters*.

the mind has a different job. Mind wants answers based on perceived facts. Mind is the meaning and identity you form about yourself and the world that reflects that identity back to you. Mind is how you formed your life and how you are within it. There is science attached to the mind. Mind exists within the brain. While mind is powerful and assists you in navigating aspects of your life, it is not as in control as it would like to think it is.

This time on earth was manifested by your Soul. With your Soul's true essence leading the way, you can more easily manage life's circumstances. Being Soul-led leads to the most suitable outcomes. You will be calmer, more present, and balanced.

This takes work. Your ego identities have developed many protective mechanisms over the course of decades on this planet. If you are locked in a regular mode of defense based on a history of having to run or fight, that work requires you to establish safety in your body. This way your inner light can more regularly lead.

I hope I am helping you break down your process and showing you ways to regularly lead with your eternal light. What manifests from Soul is better than anything you can believe. You will draw to you more Soulful experiences and people. Joy and playfulness will surround you because this is the vibration you will have.

What Soul Wants

Soul wants to be heard even through the noise of injury and doubt. Soul wants its earthly expedition. Soul wants deeper engagement in this world and is here to understand what being human feels like. Each Soul's mission and learning objectives are unique. It wants to know sensations in ways it cannot when it is not embodied. Taste, smell, and touch are profoundly human and offer up experiences like no other for your Soul.

This brilliance within is generous, considerate, gracious, knowing, and unworried. Soul exalts in a sunset or a clear, starry night. It is stirred by simple experiences: listening to a giggling infant or hearing the ominous hoot of an owl. It doesn't disregard the cyclical nature of the planet. Nor does it need it. However, it wants it. Because Soul, your Soul, wants to know this time and place.

Soul knows it's only here for a short time. This wise energy has awareness of a universal force that is greater than anything your brain or nervous system is designed to know. Soul yearns for home, for expansion, to return to its rapid-speed connection to the cosmic. But first it has work to do. Allow yourself the grounding and healing to give Soul the opportunity to do that work. Break old patterns that no longer serve you. Let your inner wisdom lead.

If you were a body without your inner light, your drives would be purely instinctual. You would only endure and not consider the effect on others. The need to survive would be a deadly one; the spoils going to the victor. Resources and the continuation of the species would be the exclusive end goal. Empathy would not exist. War would rage. Personal gain would be the only objective. Yes, I am describing much of the current state of humanity. Perhaps it is time for us to reach deeper, to seek spiritual joining by honoring the light within one another.

Calming your reactive system to make room for the wisdom within is not a weakness. It is where your strength lies. Learn to access patience for yourself and you will access patience for others. Honor the autonomous nature of your own experience and you will naturally honor that others have their own path. To prioritize your inner spirit over your fear-based responses takes work, but that work is the job your Soul wants your body to do.

Social patterns shift when we connect through calm. Human priorities change. Through the perspective of your Soul energy,

you see life as abundant and full of opportunities. You can understand others have their own struggles and challenges. You can then
create tender connection, compassion, and brilliance for others
and yourself. That energy can naturally shine outward. This is
how the world changes—through the light of your Soul.

EXERCISE
Soul Through Vagal Tone

This is an exercise that can help you deeply calm your body
to naturally experience your inner light. As I have been saying throughout the book, staying connected to your body as
you develop safety first is the way in. Notice if you dissociate,
and bring yourself back into your felt experience. Your work
in human form is to be present, aware, and compassionate—
starting with yourself first.

If you want, sit on a meditation cushion. If you have knee
or back issues, find a chair that will support your hips and back.
You will bilaterally tap in this exercise. Remember that bilateral
is left-right-left-right movement. If you would like, set a timer for
ten minutes or more, but that is not always necessary.

Through this in breath and slow chant outward, you are
engaging the throat, heart, and solar plexus chakras. These are
the energies of the upper diaphragm and ventral vagal complex. Make sure you don't get too "spacey." Stay connected to
your body as you chant, even if you need to do a slow back-
and-forth rocking movement with your body.

- Sit in an aware posture with shoulders back and feet
  on ground. This will keep you grounded in your body.

- Allow your spine and neck to be engaged by lengthening them as you sit. This makes room for the nerve fibers.
- Cross your hands over your chest in a butterfly hug. This looks like one wrist crossed over the other.
- Slowly start to tap with full palms in a one-two-one-two bilateral motion.
- As you softly tap, start an easy "ohmmm" chant.
- Make sure you don't tap too hard as you chant.
- After completing one full chant, pull in a slow breath through the nose.
- Chant on the exhale.
- Find your rhythm with chanting and bilateral tapping.
- Keep the energy of breath moving deeply into the lungs and continue with the slow exhales of chant.
- Continue this for as long as you want.
- Notice the changes in your body and emotional state as you do.
- When you stop, find a focal point in the room.
- Keep your eyes in a soft gaze.
- Sit quietly.
- Notice your breathing.
- Continue to keep the spine straight.
- Feel the breath as it flows through your nose and down into your lungs and abdomen.
- Just notice the breath as you continue to gaze.
- Notice how your body feels in a way that holds space and is curious without bringing in any shoulds or other beliefs.

- If beliefs arise, let them linger. Do not follow them. Honor that they are there and continue to keep your eyes focused.
- Just be.

I would encourage you to practice this regularly. This exercise will reset your neurobiology. It is a combination of a mindful practice and bilateral stimulation that is signaling to both hemispheres of the brain and the vagus nerve that you are safe. Build on this safety. This is how access to Soul Self begins. The more you engage in a safe, calming practice, the more easily your inner light will shine.

Don't Take Sides

Some say that if you honor your "ego" you block your ability to be "spiritual," that you either have to be spiritual or human, that life is a dichotomous, either-or experience. So many books and podcasts discuss alleviating negative thoughts, fears, and anxieties as if we can take an ice pick and chip away at these things. They state that when you get rid of the ego you reach your divinity. This puts us at such an unfair advantage and sets us up for failure—every time.

Others maintain that a perfect balance of thinking—with no diversion into the shadows—is what elevates you to the next level in the spiritual video game. If you have bad thoughts, your body will spiral into illness. Worse, some spiritual leaders claim the answer lies with them and they can lead you to some promise land if you give control over to their system of enlightenment.

But here's the thing—dichotomies take sides. In other words, if you "choose" spirituality, you disconnect from your humanness. The belief that human is bad and spirit is good creates a dualism that locks you into an everlasting battle within yourself. No one comes out alive when you won't stop fighting. Choosing sides elevates one approach over another; it creates a power dynamic within yourself. I don't know about you, but when I start working from an either-or way of thinking, I set myself up for all that anxiety and fear that people say is wrong.

Clashing internally means clashing externally. The layers of belief that we can't get it right morph into defenses. Those defenses project onto others. We start to condemn them. We compare and contrast. The internal dialogue that started as "I am not spiritual enough" becomes a projected defense of "They are not as righteous as I am." We double down into our holy books or rituals. This becomes a burdened ego.

This "if only I could alleviate my ego to be more spiritual" belief has the opposite effect. "If only" generates a sense of not being enough. "If only" says, "I haven't reached Nirvana, transcendence, or a perfect submission to factors outside of me."

"If only" sets up a rigidity in your mind that spreads outward into your daily life. It loops back to self-loathing of your ego as the barrier to spiritual awakening. The dichotomy expands.

Management of your humanness will always be at play no matter how much you are spiritually seeking. Isn't that the spiritual work?

So, what can you do differently to alleviate these dualities?

Instead of seeing life as a dichotomous, black-versus-white, or Soul-versus-human existence, I would like to propose something new. See your human experience as living in a paradoxical state. Be enquiring and accepting of the complexities of your inner world.

A paradox may appear as if it cancels itself out, but it does not. It leaves room for the unknown. It holds, with open hands, an acknowledgment of the uncertain. Like loving but dissimilar family members, paradox works to put differences aside to find common ground just so the family can be together. That is love—leaning in and leaning out, attuning to the flow with others. This is something you can learn to do. This is the movement you can apply to your inner awareness. Utilizing loving-kindness of your ego parts that reside with your Soul takes patience. It takes slowing down and accommodating in new ways. At its core, a spiritual approach to healing is a psychological one. This is the paradox.

It's a fact that to survive you must share time and space with others. As humans, community is a form of safety. You need others to share experiences and do commerce with. You feel safe when you are accepted by those you respect. You calm where you are bonded with loving people. Being with others most certainly requires adjustments. Each person generates a different response in you. Each circumstance is asking different things from you. Becoming aware of how you're connecting allows you to step back and see your experiences—and the people in them—for what they are. People then lose classification. You can be present. Intentions shift. The edges of your life soften—so does your heart.

This is how to approach your various ego parts. This is presence, where Soul can be felt.

EXERCISE
Writing Prompt: Ask the Right Questions

Spiritual growth is not about the "why." It's about the "how." Approaching your world through "how" empowers you. It helps you to draft a map for your journey by showing you a different way. Here are some questions to ask yourself.

- How do I want to be in my life?
- How do I want to experience this lifetime?
- How do I want to be with my family?

- How do I want to connect with friends?
- How do I approach my relationships in healthy ways?
- How do I get the resources I need?
- How can I get out of this mess?
- How do I heal from this broken relationship?
- How do I care for myself during this tough time?
- How do I set boundaries with others?

There may not be quick answers for you. Allow for an unfolding. Know that throughout your life these answers change as you go about things in different ways.

Human Tension Is the Spiritual Work

The most peaceful people are aware that life is contradictory. When you accept this, you can stand down from feeling as if all the complexities have to be put in order before you feel peaceful. Leaning in and leaning out—discerning what can be dealt with and what has to be left alone is freeing. Paradoxical, isn't it?

Growth as a human being has no end point. It just takes on different looks. Being in this world yet not of this world still requires you to take responsibility for the way you are in it. See your life as a journey of roads, pathways, forests, valleys, hills, and villages—certainly some mountains. But after the mountains there are still pathways; you're just in better condition to walk them.

Those mountains—a metaphor for the extremely hard times in your life—develop resiliency in you. The climb asks things of you and helps you develop psychological and spiritual maturity. The challenges are put before you to offer opportunities for new experiences. Then you get to take the strength you developed and head back down the mountain. This makes the exploration of life on the other side a little easier because you are sturdier. You have a better understanding of what you survived in life, and you can apply this to your present moment. You become a mentor, a guiding principle for those who haven't climbed yet.

Stopping in the middle of the hard parts sounds tempting at times. However, giving up brings deeper troubles. For one, you don't get to see where you would end up. Would you just pull over onto the side of the highway during a road trip and not move because you were sick of driving? Of course not. You may rest so you can resume the trip, but sitting stubbornly under the overpass brings on so many other problems and, frankly, doesn't put you in a safe place.

Heena's Story: Stopping in the Middle of the Life Road

Heena came to me because she was uncertain if she even wanted the degree she had been asked to finish by her parents. The daughter and only child of immigrants, she was the first generation to finish college. It had always been discussed that she would continue on to medical school. Her family had put a lot into her education and struggled to make ends meet at times because of their dream for her.

She reported feeling a lot of anxiety growing up because she was expected to get straight As and be the first success in the family. Now that she was finishing up her master's in infectious disease, she was expected to head to med school. Heena admitted at times she was angry but feared she would lose her parents' love if she didn't keep going. They were poor, she said, because they were putting her through school.

Lately she was spending a lot of time in bed and not going to classes. She would then scramble at the last minute to get the work done. She wasn't certain if she was acting out because of her family's expectations for her or because of her own doubts that she could do the work. At times she admitted that she was uncertain as to whether she wanted to be a doctor at all.

"I can't recall where my desire for this started. Was this my idea or theirs?" she would say regularly.

As graduation for her master's approached, Heena was waking up with panic attacks. She was pulling out the hair in her brows and in the back of her hairline so no one could see. She admitted to cutting on her thigh one day with a scalpel she took from a classroom. This scared her.

"I feel sick," she said. "I honestly don't know if med school is what I want. But I can't tell my parents."

Heena also had a history of inexplicable health issues; that seemed to be part of how she internalized stress. We had been parsing out what she wanted versus what was being expected of her. Heena liked what she was studying and found herself intrigued by how infectious diseases played a role in society but didn't know if she wanted to directly work with people.

One day, Heena came in looking disheveled and exhausted. She was three weeks from graduation. "I spent the last two weeks in bed with some guy I met at a bar. I've never smoked more pot in my life. It was really nice. I'm not sure I'm going to be able to make up the work now."

"Unprotected sex?"

She nodded, looking at once scared and pleased.

"Why?"

She shrugged.

"Is this where you want to stop? This part of the road?"

She squinted. "What do you mean?"

"Potentially pregnant by a dude you barely know? Not finishing this degree that you found interesting."

Heena was silent a while. She slumped down on my couch with both hands in her sweatshirt pockets and looked like a thirteen-year-old. I knew this personality part was leading the way and making choices for her because the rest of her was so scared.

"What do you mean by 'this part of the road'?" she asked.

"If you stop now, by having to raise a kid whose father may or may not be in the picture and smoking a shit-ton of pot to keep the anxiety at bay," I said, "you won't know what will be down the road. It's like you've just pulled your car over on the side of the highway and stopped."

Frowning, she leaned forward. "Tell me more."

"You're on a journey," I said. "We all are. This journey is one of self-discovery. If you stop now, you won't know where you will find yourself. Right now your decisions are leading you to a dead-end street."

Heena left that session in deep thought. I honestly didn't know if that metaphor was enough to get her to understand she was making choices out of fear. After that session, I didn't see her for three weeks. When she did come back, she walked in wearing her cap and gown.

"Sorry it's been a while," she said. "I had some serious catching up to do with homework."

"I can see you're happy."

She took off the cap and sat down in her shiny gown. "I went to my professors and made up the work. It was hard, but I pulled that out of my butt!" She laughed. "I also told my parents I would have to wait and see about med school."

"Really?"

"Yeah," she said. "They weren't happy, but they weren't as disappointed as I thought they would be." She leaned forward. "I also got a job at the university clinic doing research, and I'm really excited about that!"

"Incredible!"

"Oh," she said. "And I'm not pregnant. I told Mr. Pothead he had to move on."

"So, you got back into your car and started driving?"

She laughed. "Yep! And this time, I'm firmly holding the wheel."

★ ★ ★

Time on earth is a testing ground. However, life is also not a constant struggle. There is much joy, connection, happiness, and play when you seek it. Even in the hardest of lives there is pleasure and humor. Life has layers and complexity. That is what your Soul came for—to develop the paradoxical research paper you get to bring back home and assess.

Your Soul has an understanding of this journey, but it doesn't know everything. If it did, you wouldn't need new information and human experiences. You would be filling out all the answers on the exam without studying. As Dolores Cannon has said in her book *Between Death and Life*, "Life would not be a test if we knew all the answers."[128]

So, let's look at your life and the time your Soul spends here as a dwelling to be curious within. Keep your books open not out of obligation but in love. Stay inquisitive about learning. This way you have agency over how you shape this life. Set yourself up for success by letting Soul manifest the things it is asking to experience.

---

128. Cannon, *Between Life and Death*, 48.

EXERCISE
Heart Connection

The Soul amplifies love through the body. The ventral vagus complex slows your system down enough to experience that light. Here is another exercise that helps you open to heart chakra energy by tapping that vagal brake. If you are experiencing difficulties or are confused about something, just ask your heart center.

- Sit and just breathe.
- Pull connection to the heart and sit quietly.
- Connect with the sound of your heart. Hear it in your ears. Feel it beat in your chest.
- Breathe deep through your nose and slowly exhale through your mouth.
- Ask your heart the question you are struggling with.
- Let the energy of the heart speak to you.
- Allow space for anything that comes to you.

Thank any information for showing up today. Continue to just sit and connect.

Summary

Spiritual growth is not about "why" you are here but "how" you can be while you are here.

Having an ability to bounce back in situations because you can reclaim safety in your nervous system settles you onto your very right and true pathway. The most peaceful people are aware of this regular tension of being human.

To understand your egoic identities and when they are at play versus the Soul leading the way is like the loyal warriors knowing they have to stand down and let something bigger manage the external battle. This is leaning in and leaning out. This requires engagement and curiosity of your inner world.

Time on earth is a testing ground. However, life is also not a constant struggle. There is much joy, connection, happiness, and play when you seek it.

CHAPTER 10
ACCEPTANCE: THE ROAD TO HEALING

———•———

Like kindness or curiosity, healing has an intentional arc by which you can live your life. Healing might be spending long times in solitude. It might be time spent walking or reading. It might mean dinner with friends because you want to laugh and enjoy their company. Sometimes healing means pushing yourself through that exam you have to nail to get that degree or filing for divorce. Healing might be part of the aftermath of a life-changing event or choosing to take one on despite its difficulty because it is in your best interest.

Healing is not about never feeling pain again. It isn't a goal. Healing is not the perfected meditation or yoga asana or the exact right medicine. It's more about peaceful acceptance. Consider healing a moment-to-moment job, and the most powerful moments in your life are generally the simplest.

One of the outcomes to healing is being okay with not always being okay. The narrative we let roll in our heads, which may not seem very predominant at first, might be the thought you need to gently redirect. Just notice the story you are telling yourself, say hello, and change course.

When we heal past hurts, we no longer need to let them play out in our lives. We don't act out on or with others in painful ways. We are calm. We are present. We listen to ourselves and know when to be patient or to remove ourselves from those who act out and will hurt us.

Growth Means Death and Rebirth

When awareness increases and consciousness arises, you can find yourself on shaky ground. You can't go back to your old ways of being in the world. The illusions you clung to are gone. Growth puts you into a state of transition, and transitions are scary. They're the passage from one place to another, and passages are often where intimidating things happen. No longer are you the master of your own universe, the fabulous fixer, the narcissistic know-it-all, the helpless martyr, the upper-class uber-mom, the macho ladies' man, or the extroverted coach. The exterior ways of functioning fade away. The images you once cultivated are useless to you now.

Perhaps you will be forced to listen in another way. Maybe you will need to sit a while and pay attention to things differently. Maybe your thinking about something will change? Or maybe you will start to (*yikes!*) feel things. This new road of change you are on might not have a clear map, so it's natural that you will feel desperate to return to the old ways.

And, of course, there's always the possibility that something might not happen right away. Like when we have a delayed flight, we might be forced to sit and wait. Patience might have to be applied when we're much more inclined to want to run to our end goal and shout out, "Yeah, I'm spiritual now!"

Moving deeper into the subjective, less evaluative aspects of Self may mean exercising maturity in a situation we usually manipulated. Maybe it means having to end an old relationship or work situation. It might mean leaving the comforts of a hometown or a culture. It might mean learning that others are simply a mirror reflecting back at us and what we don't like in others is what we need to work on in ourselves. Ending what we know is hard. Making the effort to change is harder.

Yet, returning to the old armor we used to hide behind would be like stuffing our adult feet into a pair of sneakers we've had since middle school. Maybe we could manage to walk in them for a while, but eventually our feet would bleed from blisters, our knees would hurt from limping, and our disposition would sour because we're in pain. The domino effect of inauthenticity would wear us down, and we'd be forced to take those old shoes off.

Imagine the relief.

The space between ending something and replacing it with something new creates uncertainty and insecurity. Therapist Viktor Frankl called it "the gap between what one is and what one should become."[129]

These transitions can be the opportunity your Soul has been waiting for. If you're able to take the leap and trust that all life is about evolution, then you can find great strength. When you're on the edge of a spiritual and emotional precipice, which I'm guessing you are if you're reading this, then you can choose to have faith and leap into a new reality of change. Even if you choose to go back, you're still different.

---

129. Frankl, *Man's Search for Meaning*, 105.

EXERCISE
Writing Prompt: Releasing the Old

Think of a time you had to let go of something that was not working for you anymore. Was it a job? A relationship? A behavior? A habit? Journal about that experience. The following are some questions to help you explore that time.

- Write down something in your life you had to let go of that was hard. What was it?
- Did you let go easily? Did you fight the transition?
- Were you scared?
- What was the fear (e.g., being left alone or not knowing how else to "be")?
- Did you feel frustration at having to change?
- Did you see yourself as a victim?
- Did you get angry?
- How did you release the old pattern?
- What helped you?
- Were you able to work toward a point of acceptance?
- How did you change and grow?
- What did you learn about yourself after releasing the old?

If applicable, explore the following questions instead.

- Do you still hang on to an old pattern (like returning to an old relationship when you need to disconnect)?
- If you know this old pattern hurts you, what keeps you returning to it? Why?

Return to this exercise when you are feeling uncertain about change in your life.

Transitions

Each life transition has an aspect of mourning to it. Those transitions can be considered good or bad. If you cannot mourn the loss of your divorce, your child going off to school, having left an old city for a new one or one job for the another, then you can't fully embrace this next phase of growth. When you marry, you leave one state of being for another. If you don't accept this transition from singlehood to couple-hood, you waver in your commitment to the marriage.

Mourning is an active verb. It is the intentional act of working through a loss. Mourning a divorce may require trusting that this place in time will lead you to understand more about yourself. Mourning may look like going to therapy, journaling, talking it out with friends, practicing self-care, or having a good cry. Mourning itself is the transition, but because mourning requires feeling the loss, we tend to avoid this part. Actively mourning is not about keeping you in a place of sadness and uncertainty. When you engage in the loss, regardless of how big or small, you're moving through with intent. Mourning is what brings you to the other side. Denying the effect change has on you keeps you stuck in the past. Being present to your needs—the pleasant as well as the difficult ones—brings you to your new normal. In the acceptance of the loss, you're able to integrate its meaning so that you can continue forward movement.

Once you grow, going back to your previous state of being is more painful than before. It is the universal law of growth. A seed once planted and sprouted must continue on a path of growth lest it wither. It can never return to its state as a seed. And if it allows itself to thrive, it can produce more seeds and follow its natural course of being.

Getting to Peace

Part of being human is acceptance of your Soul's choice to stay in a human body. This means having a loving reception of what is happening. This helps you respect just how hard your flesh, blood, and nervous system work to keep you here. Befriending and welcoming this human self of yours can be a lot of work depending on how unsafe you have experienced your life as being.

Soul wants healing from old experiences that have created injury. It wants forgiveness and resolution with people who instilled pain because, frankly, it wants to keep rolling down the highway and experience the sites along the way. Body wants protections and guarantees that bad things won't happen on that road again.

The term *trauma* gets bandied about these days as a household word. This is not a bad thing since the world needs a wider discussion about how to live safer. However, like any term that gets overexposed, it gets watered down and loses its initial impact. Trauma is anything we experience that is out of a normal range of safety. When you live with trauma, you struggle with discerning if you are safe in your present circumstances. You lose your sense of peace.

EXERCISE
Writing Prompt: Thanking the Voices Inside Your Head

We are so inclined to shut down the voices inside of our head that are too loud and overbearing. Sometimes we do this by finding distractions, sometimes by numbing. Neither approach is long term nor effective.

Interestingly, it's not Soul wanting to shut anything out; it's other voices. Like a regular loop of arguments from a battling family, those voices can intensify and lock us down.

As I hope you have learned through much of my work, leaning into the discomfort in your body is really the only way through. This is the same for the dialogues in our head.

If you can see this conflicting stream of information as little children all vying for attention at once, does that help you? Imagine you are sitting on the floor of a day care center listening to a lot of children. Know they believe they have been left alone for a long time and are rushing toward you to fill you in on what is happening.[130] They all have different views about being left alone, and they are all different ages.

- Take your journal and pencils and be ready to draw or write.
- Listen to one voice.
- Notice what that voice is saying. Write it down.
- See if you can attach a child, form, or color to that voice.
- Let this image know you are hearing it.
- Now see if you can notice another voice.
- Listen to what it wants you to know and write it down.
- See if you can attach a form, color, shape, or movement to that voice.
- Honor what it is telling you.
- Thank it for showing up.

Getting to Congruency

Creating from the Soul is about being congruent. Being congruent within yourself means being the same on the inside as you are on the outside. Congruency is authenticity. It is about leading from

---

130. Schwartz and Sweezy, *Internal Family Systems Therapy*, 132.

your inner being. When you are in your Soul energy, you are being congruent. Your genuineness is present. Congruency means the world experiences your internal luster, gentle strength, and capacity to be centered.

If you fear that leading from your internal light is too vulnerable, you may still be thinking from your defensives. The essence of who you are cannot be hurt. It cannot be twisted to fulfill someone else's insecure agenda. The strongest people in the world are leading from this essence within themselves. They are calm, aware, gracious, centered, and understanding that life and the people in it change.

In geometry congruency refers to two objects having the same shape or size. For us humans, congruency isn't about matching another's shape and size but deeply knowing our own. Being psychologically congruent means being consistent or compatible within oneself. Congruency means knowing who you are, what feels right for you, how to honor this connection within yourself, and leaving others to their own journey.

If congruency is the only concept that you take away from this book, then you are doing well. This is because congruency takes being honest with yourself, knowing what you need to heal, and reconciling maladaptive beliefs that you have to protect your Soul Self. It takes intention to be kind and balanced first with yourself, then with others.

To be congruent means to heal. To be Soul-led means to trust in the intention of that healing. Living congruently also means having a life that reflects this. It also means at times we have to weigh factors within our lives that may seem incongruent. A good example might be the person who dislikes their job. Do they stay and complain because they fear they will never find another job?

Do they have choices to find something else to pay their bills? Or perhaps they have a family relying on them. Staying at the job to support the thing that means more to them—their family—might be the most congruent choice for them.

Balancing priorities is something you will always have to work through. Being as congruent as you can be while you are doing this is working from your Soul.

Getting to Creation

Creating from your Soul is manifestation. It is calming your system enough to allow the gracious energy within to lead. When this happens, you live your truth. Life becomes an experience of trust and presence. Wisdom can be ridiculously simple, yet it feels wildly out of reach at times.

Have you ever been exactly where you need to be, doing the absolute thing you need to be doing? Have you noticed that when this happens all your problems seem to find resolution? Things just work out right. The energy in your body feels in alignment when you drop down into you. What you need is suddenly there. You feel safe.

There is equanimity when you operate from the place of calm and higher knowing. Even in the hard times, the next right step, word, or act that is done from a place of honesty and grace can change everything for you. This is Soul-creation.

If everyone on this earthly plane understood they have this perfect illumination within and they could allow it to lead, humanity would be much further along. Soul-creation gives you a higher perspective about life. It allows you to honor the light in others without giving way to fear. Famine, hatred, and violence do not manifest from Soul; they manifest from a perception of lack.

Your Soul is here to do the next right thing. It is doing the best for you. It wants harmony so you have room to move. It wants peace so you can live well. It wants safe connection for your body and psyche so you can feel and express love. These are not lofty pursuits.

Soul-creation is your highest energy at work. When this energy within is the major influencer, life becomes vivid. Things work out the way they are supposed to. Life just feels right. To create from the Soul takes a management of your human system in loving, patient ways.

The word *creation* in this sense is not always intended as an action word. Creating can be what we experience when we are still. Creation is the energy we naturally produce through our Soul. We can be actively engaging or be in stillness. Life is a bit like a hologram of reality either way.[131] We create our own reality.

Getting to Simple Joys

Life will always throw us conflict, defeat, and disturbances. Even if these problems are not humanly designed, we have natural disasters, death, and painful accidents. This is the uncertainty of living on this earth. Many things can't be controlled—only managed.

The objective of spiritually thriving as a human comes down to acceptance. Acceptance of the past. Acceptance of the loss. Acceptance that people cannot be controlled nor should be. Acceptance that you have your own free will. Acceptance that you are responsible for your own actions. Acceptance that you are responsible for your own healing.

---

131. Laszlo, *Reconnecting to the Source.*

Getting to joy is working with acceptance. When we do this, we stop writhing in frustration that things are not what we want them to be. When we are still and seeing things for what they are, we can take the time to find the glimmers. A dear friend who had experienced the loss of a loved one told me once that during the darkest times of her grief, she sought comfort in the little things.

We cannot make everything outside of us quiet and calm. That power lies within. It is a mighty power. When we know that the only thing within our control is ourselves, we can access joy.

Sam's Story: Pain, Turned to Kindness, Turned to Forgiveness

Sam is a client that I have been working with for years. Because of his father's heavy addiction to alcohol when Sam was growing up, he struggled to find any calm in his life. After years of family fights that always ended in Sam being beaten by a drunken father, Sam struggled with PTSD.

The father eventually left the family. When Sam was sixteen and out driving around with friends, he spied his father sleeping in a park. The father was wearing a rugby shirt Sam had bought him years earlier. Sam was devastated and sick to his stomach. He never told his mother, who was scrambling to keep the family together by working two jobs. He feared she might go find him and attempt to "prop him up and make him be normal" like Sam said she always did.

"She's working her ass off, and he's partying with his cheap beers in the park." His bitterness was understandable.

Until we started doing therapy, Sam could barely find words to describe his pain. Instead, he would lean into his rage as a way to push back against any emotional vulnerability.

"He was the worst example of a man to me. A coward," Sam would say. "I can never forgive him."

As so many children who grew up with underfunctioning alcoholic parents do, Sam overcompensated by achieving success. When your parent is not providing basic needs, this can be a way out of living below the poverty line. Sam put himself through college and law school. He now works as a successful lawyer at a health insurance agency.

What brought Sam to counseling was his inability to maintain a lasting, loving relationship. He was also noticing the more stress he was under at work, the shorter his temper was getting. The one thing Sam was not going to risk was his career.

Sam chose not to drink because he didn't want to be like his father, however he struggled with not judging others when they got drunk. Through our work, he was able to see how scared he got around someone who drank too much.

"Yeah," he admitted. "Watching people lose their ability to manage themselves is a trigger for me."

It took some time in our work to help him understand that not imbibing in the drug of choice that your parent had did not mean you escaped the addiction dance. Sam's drugs were success and rage. Through trauma work and helping him understand the addictive cycle in families, Sam was able to access more internal balance and insight. He attended weekly meditation groups and was in a relationship that was going on eight months. Sam's biggest struggle was the rage he felt when he saw an elderly homeless man on the street.

"Still makes me sick to my stomach."

This was the one EMDR trauma target Sam's defenses would allow us to go deeper with. That night he saw his father in the park was so overwhelming he feared processing it. So, we went slow around it.

One night, after a long day of work, Sam decided to get takeout for dinner. As he was standing in line at the counter to pick up the food, the man in front of him was struggling to pay.

"His card kept declining," Sam said. "Then I smelled that twinge of alcohol on him, and my stomach just churned."

I nodded.

"But"—Sam lifted a finger and raised a brow—"I decided to work my dharma and apply all the skills you and I have been working on."

"And?" I smiled and learned forward.

"I first needed to ground myself because I could feel myself dissociating. The guy kinda looked like my dad, you know, that regular drunk-old-man look."

"Oh?" I laughed.

"While I was grounding in my breath, I watched the guy leave," he said. "I thought maybe he was just getting a beer while waiting for his food and that's why he smelled. Then I saw him walk outside. He wasn't wearing a coat, and he leaned down and picked up an old, dirty backpack." Sam paused. "Something washed over me. I dunno. You've turned me into an old softy or something."

We both laughed.

"I told the guy behind the bar to put the man's food on my bill."

"Seriously?"

Sam nodded. "Yeah, I ran out and handed him his food. I even made it a point of looking him in the eyes when I did it."

"Woah."

"He had that old alcoholic stare that my dad had." Sam nodded. "This time I wasn't freaked out, though. And guess what?"

"What?"

"I gave him my freakin' coat!"

I laughed. "Literally gave him the coat off your back?"

Sam tried to laugh but choked up a bit. He drew in a deep breath. "But you know what? That wasn't the half of it. Something in that was a milestone for me, right? With my trauma, right?"

I nodded.

"But what happened next is what actually made me cry." He smiled. "The guy from the restaurant was outside standing behind me holding my food. He told me that what I just did was the nicest thing he had ever seen anyone do."

"Wow."

"The restaurant dude said he was never going to forget what he saw me do. He was choked up." Sam looked at me for a long time. "It was an unintentional metta thing. What I did for that homeless guy was me trying to overcome my old stuff. I had no idea I would be sending loving-kindness to others in the process."

Over the next few sessions, we discussed Sam's father's trauma growing up. Sam's grandfather had beaten Sam's father until he was unconscious. That cycle had been repeating, perhaps for generations.

"And he didn't have a trauma therapist to work with," Sam said.

"Yes," I said. "Do you have any new understandings around your father since you've been doing your own work?"

"I wonder if he left to keep things from getting any worse?" Sam took in a deep breath. "I suppose we will never know."

"Maybe," I said. "But does that belief bring you comfort? Does it feel likely?"

"Yeah," Sam said. "When he was sober, he was a sweet guy. Maybe something deeper in him was trying to protect me in his own weird way."

Sam eventually drove back around the park where he had seen his father two decades earlier. There was no sign of him. Sam also started to bring blankets, jackets, and other resources to the people he would see sleeping in that park. He had even called the authorities to see if his father might have been arrested or found dead. Given that many homeless people whose identities are not clear get buried in an unmarked grave, Sam would never know if his father was dead or had moved to another town.

"I suppose I can fill in the blanks. He can become part of my own story of forgiveness," Sam said. "The only thing I can control is to send out Metta Prayers to those that are struggling."

Metta Prayer

The Metta Prayer is also known as the Loving-Kindness Meditation. The word *metta* is Pali for "loving-kindness" or "benevolence." It is a traditional Buddhist prayer that is intended to cultivate unconditional love and compassion—first toward oneself and then to others.

The practice of using the Metta Prayer involves silently repeating phrases that express good wishes and intentions for oneself and others. I leave you with this Metta Prayer. I first wish you loving-kindness on your journey, and I hope you use this prayer for your own self as you spread loving-kindness to others.

> *May I be filled with loving-kindness.*
> *May I be happy and healthy.*
> *May I feel connected and calm.*
> *May I be free from suffering.*
> *May I live in peace.*

~

May you be filled with loving-kindness.
May you be happy and healthy.
May you feel connected and calm.
May you be free from suffering.
May you live in peace.

~

May all be filled with loving-kindness.
May all be happy and healthy.
May all feel connected and calm.
May all be free from suffering.
May all live in peace.

My Soul honors your Soul on this journey of life. Be well. Heed your physical as well as your emotional experiences. Walk with intention and care. When you trip, remember it is just a moment along your way. Get up, brush yourself off, and know there are good things ahead. Namaste.

CONCLUSION

———•———

You come to earth and join with a human body to learn. As you travel along your life journey, your Soul knowledge increases and becomes more aware. The Soul parts aren't so hard. They shine through in moments of grace and love. Soul initiates connection with others to laugh or feel hopeful. It's the human parts that get confusing and scary.

The vagus nerve and the brain, along with the connecting organs of the heart and lungs, the digestive system, and the musculoskeletal structure, make up a complex communication system. Not only do they perform the basic functions of metabolizing food, reproducing, and finding a balance to keep you alive, but they also register threats from outside of you. In normal times, it's easy to be spiritually connected because you feel safe. In disrupted times, the body's defense mechanisms kick in. If those defenses get too dysregulated, it feels nearly impossible to listen to your inner wisdom.

My discussion of the vagus nerve through polyvagal theory and how your autonomic nervous system keeps you safe is intended to help you differentiate what is an emotional or spiritual experience versus a neurobiological response. Learning this difference takes the shame out of your views about yourself. Shame is not derived from Soul. Shame can block your ability to connect to your light and the light of others. Shame is a learned message that something is wrong with you. There is nothing wrong with you. There is only your free will and an opportunity to work beyond the pain you are in.

Your chakras and vagus nerve are extensions of each other. Chakra energy is the etheric energy of your Soul as it negotiates and emanates from the branches of your nervous system. I see the seven main chakras as seven dimensions of your human psychological experience. Together they work as a guidance tool that, when heeded, will direct you along the road of life.

In my view, the chakras have various psychological dimensions to them and align with all three branches of the vagus nerve: ventral, sympathetic, and dorsal. Those dimensions are your experience with your body, or root chakra; your early childhood emotions, or sacral chakra; your mind and how it forms identities, or your solar plexus chakra; your ability to feel compassion for self and others, or your heart chakra; your ability to connect with others through words and sound, or your throat chakra; your spiritual and imaginal inner world, or your third eye chakra; and your universal connection to experience empathy, or your crown chakra.

Your vagus nerve, like your brain, is bilateral. It means there is a left and a right side. There are three states of safety your vagus nerve experiences according to Porges's polyvagal theory. The first state is immobility, and it derives from the dorsal vagal nerve complex. The second state is mobility, which is activated from the sympathetic branch. The third state is safety. This is through the ventral vagal complex, which connects to your heart, lungs, and throat. These three nerve branches play distinct roles in helping you navigate your world.

Thank your body for how it works to protect you. Learn to recognize when it might be doing its job a little too well by registering a lack of safety when there is none or not registering safety when it needs to. Be kind to your body. Be inquisitive about your nervous system and the history stored in it. Find a more neutral presence. Remember that curiosity of what is happening in the moment is what helps you experience equanimity.

Be good to yourself and that includes physically taking care of your body. In doing so, you can be good to others. Heart, lung, and digestive health are vagus nerve health. This will create that ripple effect that is needed to change a larger pattern in the world. Small steps, kind intention, and healing are the ways forward.

Never forget that your life is a journey that you get to experience. It's a balancing act of human survival instincts and Soulful insights. If you can remember this through the times of pain, disruption, disharmony, and general slogging in the mundane, you can approach the experience from a perspective of personal ownership and power. Life has brilliant moments. Then there are the small steps—again. Through it all, be compassionate to yourself and others. Remember the people next to you in line, walking down the street, or working alongside you are also Souls here to learn.

ACKNOWLEDGMENTS

W riting the acknowledgments in your book is like saving the best for last. As my work has expanded, some wonderful new people appeared in my life to help get this healing message out. Then there are the ones who have always been there. I thank two dear friends who have been through multiple versions of multiple manuscripts throughout our decades together. My heart always goes out to Celeste Bradley, who has been a friend and co-creator along this life path and has dragged me to the finish line in thought, word, and sometimes deed more than once, and Dr. Ann Clark, who has also been a writing partner as well as a mutual spiritual warrior, always seeking and wanting to understand the plan of the universe. I would also like to thank Victoria Henderson, another friend over the decades, who worked me through the technical overwhelm; Dr. Rosa Serra, who helped with anatomy questions; Mary Kay and Hannah Morgan; and the Llewellyn team, which is more than a pleasure to work with. So happy we got the band back together for this book! I'd like to acknowledge David Smith and Stephanie Naman, for their friendship and creative support, and Carolyn Nemeth, my beach earthing co-researcher. Thank you to my longtime friends for all the birthday and cycling parties, who have no idea what I write about but listen to me go on in great detail about it anyway, and to my son, Davis, one of the great anchors in my life. Stay connected, dear reader. CJLlewelyn.com.

RESOURCES

•————————•

Finding the Right Professional for Trauma Processing

I cannot stress enough that you find a licensed therapist with either a master's degree or PhD who is also trauma informed. Licensure indicates the professional has met certain educational and training qualifications. Just like doctors, mental health providers all have similar education but beyond their degrees, they pursue various specialties and training skills.

Discussions in the general public about trauma are increasing (as they should). This empowers people to understand their past and how their bodies and perceptions have been shaped by traumatic incidences. As this subject becomes more popular, so should clarification of who the proper professionals are to help. Helping a client relieve traumatic responses requires a base of knowledge that extends beyond being trauma informed. Licensed mental health professionals have knowledge about attachment styles, organic issues, and foundations in theories. Most importantly, licensure boards hold therapists to ethical standards. Therapists are expected to update their training through continuing education units and seek consults with other professionals.

Life coaches that refer to themselves as trauma coaches come from various backgrounds. Unless they have a qualified master's degree or PhD in a mental health field, they have no framework in pathologies or other important therapeutic underpinnings. Some neuro-experiential trainings are not available to anyone that does not have at least a master's degree and are pursing licensure. That does not mean life coaches aren't an added benefit to the helping community. Many are also licensed mental health providers which is the perfect combination as each approach has separate goals.

Further Reading

Energy Work

Hands of Light: A Guide to Healing Through the Human Energy Field by Barbara Ann Brennan

Infinite Mind: Science of the Human Vibrations of Consciousness by Valerie V. Hunt

The Reiki Manual: A Training Guide for Reiki Students, Practitioners, and Masters by Penelope Quest

The Serpent Power: The Secrets of Tantric & Shaktic Yoga by Arthur Avalon

Why Woo-Woo Works: The Surprising Science Behind Meditation, Reiki, Crystals, and Other Alternative Practices by David R. Hamilton

Health of the Vagus Nerve

Accessing the Healing Power of the Vagus Nerve: Self-Help Exercises for Anxiety, Depression, Trauma, and Autism by Stanley Rosenburg

Anchored: How to Befriend Your Nervous System Using Polyvagal Theory by Deb Dana, LCSW

The Brainbow Blueprint: A Clinical Guide to Integrative Medicine and Nutrition for Mental Well-Being by Leslie Korn

Nutrition Essentials for Mental Health: A Complete Guide to the Food-Mood Connection by Leslie Korn

Polyvagal Practices: Anchoring the Self in Safety by Deb Dana

Internal Family Systems

Internal Family Systems for Shame and Guilt by Martha Sweezy

Internal Family Systems Therapy for Addictions: Trauma-Informed, Compassion-Based Interventions for Substance Use, Eating, Gambling and More by Cece Sykes

Outshining Trauma: A New Vision of Radical Self-Compassion Integrating Internal Family Systems and Buddhist Meditation by Ralph De La Rosa

Somatic Internal Family Systems Therapy: Awareness, Breath, Resonance, Movement, and Touch in Practice by Susan McConnell

Transcending Trauma: Healing Complex PTSD with Internal Family Systems Therapy by Frank G. Anderson

Mindfulness

Don't Tell Me to Relax: Emotional Resilience in the Age of Rage, Feels, and Freak-Outs by Ralph De La Rosa

Mindfulness: A Practical Guide to Awakening by Joseph Goldstein

The Miracle of Mindfulness: An Introduction to the Practice of Meditation by Thich Nhat Hanh

Mindfulness for Beginners: Reclaiming the Present Moment—and Your Life by Jon Kabat-Zinn

Mindfulness in Plain English by Bhante Gunaratana

The Mindful Way Through Depression: Freeing Yourself from Chronic Unhappiness by Mark Williams, John Teasdale, Zindel Segal and Jon Kabat-Zinn

The Monkey Is the Messenger: Meditation and What Your Busy Mind Is Trying to Tell You by Ralph De La Rosa

Training the Mind and Cultivating Loving-Kindness by Chögyam Trungpa

Trauma

The Complex PTSD Treatment Manual: An Integrative, Mind-Body Approach to Trauma Recovery by Arielle Schwartz

It Didn't Start With You: How Inherited Family Trauma Shapes Who We Are and How to End the Cycle by Mark Wolynn

The Post-Traumatic Growth Guidebook: Practical Mind-Body Tools to Heal Trauma, Foster Resilience, and Awaken Your Potential by Arielle Schwartz

Transforming the Living Legacy of Trauma: A Workbook for Survivors and Therapists by Janina Fisher

Trauma and the 12 Steps: An Inclusive Guide to Enhancing Recovery by Jamie Marich

What My Bones Know: A Memoir of Healing from Complex Trauma by Stephanie Foo

BIBLIOGRAPHY

Ainsworth, Mary D. Salter, Mary C. Blehar, Everett Waters, and Sally Wall. *Patterns of Attachment: A Psychological Study of the Strange Situation*. Lawrence Erlbaum Associates, 1978.

Alexander, Eben. *Proof of Heaven: A Neurosurgeon's Journey into the Afterlife*. Simon & Schuster, 2012.

Allen, Jon G. *Coping with Trauma: Hope through Understanding*. American Psychiatric Publishing, 2005.

Al Alawi, Abdullah M, Sandawana William Majoni, and Henrik Falhammar. "Magnesium and Human Health: Perspectives and Research Directions." *International Journal of Endocrinology* 2018, no. 1: (April 2018). https://doi.org/10.1155/2018/9041694.

Ali, Muzaffar, Jose Carlos Pachon Maetos, Asim Kichloo et al. "Management Strategies for Vasovagal Syncope." *PACE: Pacing and Clinical Electrophysiology* 44, no. 12 (November 2021): 2100–2108. https://doi.org/10.1111/pace.14402.

Avalon, Arthur. *The Serpent Power: The Secrets of Tantric and Shakti Yoga*. Revised Edition. Dover Publications, 2023.

Aydin, Muhammet Ali, Tushar V Salkukhe, Iris Wilke et al. "Management and Therapy of Vasovagal Syncope: A Review." *World Journal of Cardiology* 2, no. 10 (October 2010): 308–15.

Batchelor, Stephen. *After Buddhism: Rethinking the Dharma for a Secular Age*. Yale University Press, 2015.

Beck, Judith S. *Cognitive Behavioral Therapy: Basics and Beyond*. 3rd ed. Guilford Press, 2020.

Begum, Jabeen. "Top Foods High in Choline." November 22, 2022. https://www.webmd.com/diet/foods-high-in-choline.

Bello-Morales, Raquel, Sabina Andreu, and José Antonio López-Guerrero. "The Role of Herpes Simplex Virus Type 1 Infection in Demyelination of the Central Nervous System." *International Journal of Molecular Sciences* 21, no. 14 (July 2020): 5026.

Berlant, Lauren. *Cruel Optimism*. Duke University Press, 2011.

Bodhi, Bhikkhu. *The Noble Eightfold Path: Way to the End of Suffering*. BPS Pariyatti Editions, 2020.

Bowen, Sarah, Neha Chawla, and G. Alan Marlatt. *Mindfulness-Based Relapse Prevention for Addictive Behaviors: A Clinician's Guide*. Guilford Press, 2010.

Bowlby, John. *Attachment*. Vol. 1 of *Attachment and Loss*. Basic Books, 1969.

Brach, Tara. *Trusting the Gold: Uncovering Your Natural Goodness*. Sounds True, 2021.

Brooks, Kelly, and Jg Carter. "Overtraining, Exercise, and Adrenal Insufficiency." *Journal of Novel Physiotherapies* 3, no. 125 (February 2013):11717. https://doi.org/10.4172/2165-7025.1000125.

Brown, Brené. *I Thought It Was Just Me (But It Isn't): Making the Journey from "What Will People Think?" to "I Am Enough."* Avery, 2007.

Cannon, Dolores. *Between Death and Life*. Ozark Mountain Publishing, 2013.

Chae, Kwon-Seok, Soo-Chan Kim, Hye-Jin Kwon, and Yongkuk Kim. "Human Magnetic Sense Is Mediated by a Light and Magnetic Field Resonance-Dependent Mechanism." *Scientific Reports* 12, no. 8997 (May 2022). https://doi.org/10.1038/s41598-022-12460-6.

Chevalier, Gaétan, and Stephen T. Sinatra. "Emotional Stress, Heart Rate Variability, Grounding, and Improved Autonomic Tone: Clinical Applications." *Integrative Medicine* 10, no. 3 (June/July 2011): 16–21.

Chozen Bays, Jan. *Mindful Eating: A Guide to Rediscovering a Healthy and Joyful Relationship with Food*. Shambala Publications, 2009.

Dale, Cyndi. *The Subtle Body: An Encyclopedia of Your Energetic Anatomy*. Sounds True, 2009.

Damasio, Antonio R. *Descartes' Error: Emotion, Reason, and the Human Brain*. Putman, 1994.

Dana, Deb. *Anchored: How to Befriend Your Nervous System Using Polyvagal Theory*. Sounds True, 2021.

Dana, Deb. *The Polyvagal Theory in Therapy: Engaging the Rhythm of Regulation*. W. W. Norton, 2018.

de Baaij, Jeroen H. F., Joost G. J. Hoenderop, and René J. M. Bindels. "Magnesium in Man: Implications for Health and Disease." *Physiological Reviews* 95, no. 1 (January 2015): 1–46. https://doi.org/10.1152/physrev.00012.2014.

De La Rosa, Ralph. *The Monkey Is the Messenger: Meditation and What Your Busy Mind Is Trying to Tell You*. Shambala, 2019.

Descartes, René. *Discourse on Method*. Macmillan, 1986.

"Diaphragmatic Breathing." Cleveland Clinic. Updated March 30, 2022. https://my.clevelandclinic.org/health/articles/9445 -diaphragmatic-breathing.

"Diabetes Statistics." National Institute of Diabetes and Digestive and Kidney Diseases. Accessed January 4, 2025. https:// www.niddk.nih.gov/health-information/health-statistics /diabetes-statistics.

Emoto, Masaru. *The Hidden Messages in Water*. Atria Books, 2001.

"Energetic Communication." In *Science of the Heart*. HeartMath Institute. https://www.heartmath.org/research/science -of-the-heart/energetic-communication/.

Epstein, Mark. *The Trauma of Everyday Life*. Penguin Books, 2014.

Evans, Patricia. *Controlling People: How to Recognize, Understand, and Deal with People Who Try to Control You*. Adams Media, 2003.

Feldenkrais, Moshe. *The Elusive Obvious: The Convergence of Movement, Neuroplasticity, and Health*. North Atlantic Books, 2017.

Felten, David L., Michael K. O'Banion, and Mary Summo Maida. *Netter's Atlas of Neuroscience*. 4th ed. Elsevier, 2022.

Fisher, Janina. *Healing the Fragmented Selves of Trauma Survivors: Overcoming Internal Self-Alienation*. Routledge/Taylor & Francis Group, 2017.

Frankl, Viktor E. *Man's Search for Meaning*. Beacon Press, 2006.

Friedman, Matthew J., Terence M. Keane, and Patricia A. Resick, eds. *Handbook of PTSD: Science and Practice*. Guilford Press, 2010.

Grand, David. *Brainspotting: The Revolutionary New Therapy for Rapid and Effective Change.* Sounds True, 2013.

Goldstein, Joseph. *Mindfulness: A Practical Guide to Awakening.* Sounds True, 2016.

Goldstein, Joseph, and Jack Kornfield. *Seeking the Heart of Wisdom: The Path of Insight Meditation.* Shambala Press, 2001.

Gunaratana, Bhante. *Mindfulness in Plain English.* Wisdom Publications, 2011.

Guo, Y. P., J. G. McLeod, and J. Baverstrock. "Pathological Changes in the Vagus Nerve in Diabetes and Chronic Alcoholism." *Journal of Neurology, Neurosurgery, and Psychiatry* 50, no. 11 (1987): 1449–53.

Hanson, Rick, and Richard Mendius. *Buddha's Brain: The Practical Neuroscience of Happiness, Love & Wisdom.* New Harbinger Publications, 2009.

Hayes, Stephen C., Kirk D. Strosahl, and Kelly G. Wilson. *Acceptance and Commitment Therapy: The Process and Practice of Mindful Change.* Guilford Press, 2016.

Harwood, John L. "Polyunsaturated Fatty Acids: Conversion to Lipid Mediators, Roles in Inflammatory Diseases and Dietary Sources." *International Journal of Molecular Sciences* 24, no. 10 (May 2023): 8838. https://doi.org/10.3390/ijms24108838.

Hui, Li, and Amanda J. Page. "Altered Vagal Signaling and Its Pathophysiological Roles in Functional Dyspepsia." *Frontiers in Neuroscience* 16 (April 2022). https://doi.org/10.3389/fnins.2022.858612.

Hunt, Valerie V. *Infinite Mind: Science of the Human Vibrations of Consciousness.* Echo Point Books & Media, 2023.

Husebye, Eystein S., Simon H. Pearce, Nils P. Krone et al. "Adrenal Insufficiency." *Lancet* 397, no. 10274 (February 2021): 613–29. https://doi.org/10.1016/S0140-6736(21)00136-7.

Jabs, Harry, and Beverly Rubik. "Detecting Subtle Energies with a Physical Sensor Array." *Cosmos and History: The Journal of Natural and Social Philosophy* 15, no. 1 (2019): 171–92.

Jelusich, Richard. *Eye of the Lotus: Psychology of the Chakras*. Lotus Press, 2004.

Jin, Hao, Mengtong Li, Eric Jeong et al. "A Body–Brain Circuit that Regulates Body Inflammatory Responses." *Nature* 630 (2024): 695–703. https://doi.org/10.1038/s41586-024-07469-y

Judith, Anodea. *Eastern Body, Western Mind: Psychology and the Chakra System as a Path of the Self*. Celestial Arts, 1996.

Jung, C. G. *Archetypes and the Collective Unconscious*. Volume 9, part 1 of *The Collected Works of C. G. Jung*, edited by Gerhard Adler and R. F. C. Hull. Princeton University Press, 1969.

Jung, C. G. *Man and His Symbols*. Doubleday, 1964.

Jung, C. G. *The Red Book: A Reader's Edition*. Edited by Sonu Shamdasani. W. W. Norton, 2012.

Kabat-Zinn, Jon. *Full Catastrophe Living: Using the Wisdom of Your Body and Mind to Face Stress, Pain, and Illness*. Bantam Books, 2013.

Kabat-Zinn, Jon. "Mindfulness-Based Interventions in Context: Past, Present, and Future." *Clinical Psychology Science and Practice* 10, no. 2 (2003): 144–56.

Kabat-Zinn, Jon. *Wherever You Go, There You Are: Mindfulness Meditation in Everyday Life: A Guide to Your Place in the Universe and an Inquiry into Who and What You Are*. Hachette Go, 2023.

Kansakar, Urna, Valentina Trimarco, Pasquale Mone, Fahimeh Varzideh, Angela Lombardi, and Gaetano Santulli. "Choline Supplements: An Update." *Frontiers in Endocrinology* 14 (March 2023). https://doi.org/10.3389/fendo.2023.1148166.

Khalid, Sidra, Shahid Bashir, Riffat Mehboob et al. "Effects of Magnesium and Potassium Supplementation on Insomnia and Sleep Hormones in Patients with Diabetes Mellitus." *Frontiers in Endocrinology* 15 (October 2024). https://doi.org/10.3389/fendo.2024.1370733.

Korn, Leslie. *The Brainbow Blueprint: A Clinical Guide to Integrative Medicine and Nutritional Mental Well Being*. PESI Publishing, 2023.

Korn, Leslie. *Nutrition Essentials for Mental Health: A Complete Guide to the Food Mood Connection*. W. W. Norton, 2016.

Kornfield, Jack. *The Wise Heart: A Guide to the Universal Teachings of Buddhist Psychology*. Bantam Books, 2008.

Koyuncu, Orkide O., Ian B. Hogue, and Lynn W. Enquist. "Virus Infections in the Nervous System." *Cell Host Microbe* 13, no. 4 (April 2013): 379–93. https://doi.org/10.1016/j.chom.2013.03.010.

Lanius, Ulrich F., Sandra L. Paulsen, and Frank M. Corrigan, eds. *Neurobiology and Treatment of Traumatic Dissociation: Towards an Embodied Self*. Springer Publishing Company, 2014.

Laszlo, Ervin. *Reconnecting to Source: The New Science of Spiritual Experience, How It Can Change You, and How It Can Transform the World*. St. Martin's Essentials, 2020.

LeDoux, Joseph. *The Emotional Brain: The Mysterious Underpinnings of the Emotional Life*. Simon & Schuster, 1996.

Linehan, Marsha. *DBT Skills Training Handouts and Worksheets*. Second Edition. Guilford Press, 2014.

Levine, Peter A. *Waking the Tiger: Healing Trauma: The Innate Capacity to Transform Overwhelming Experiences*. North Atlantic Books, 1997.

Li, Ruiyun, Zhiyuan Li, Yi Huang, Kaiyan Hu, Bin Ma, and Yuan Yang. "The Effect of Magnesium Alone or Its Combination with Other Supplements on the Markers of Inflammation, OS and Metabolism in Women with Polycystic Ovarian Syndrome (PCOS): A Systematic Review." *Frontiers in Endocrinology* 13 (August 2022). https://doi.org/10.3389/fendo.2022.974042.

Littleton, John M. "Alcohol, the Vagus Nerve, and Multi-Organ Inflammation." University of Kentucky. https://grantome .com/grant/NIH/R21-AA020188-01.

Llewelyn, C. J., *Chakras and the Vagus Nerve: Tap into the Healing Combination of Subtle Energy & Your Nervous System*. Llewellyn Publications, 2023.

Loper, Hailley, Monique Leinen, Logan Bassoff et al. "Both High Fat and High Carbohydrate Diets Impair Vagus Nerve Signaling of Satiety." *Science Reports* 11, no. 1 (May 2021): 10394. https://doi.org/10.1038/s41598-021-89465-0.

Mao, Tianxin, Bowen Guo, and Hengyi Rao. "Unraveling the Complex Interplay between Insomnia, Anxiety, and Brain Networks." *Sleep* 47, no. 3 (March 2024): zsad330. https://doi.org/10.1093/sleep/zsad330.

Mayer, Emeran. *The Mind-Gut Connection: How the Hidden Conversation within Our Bodies Impacts Our Mood, Our Choices, and Our Overall Health.* HarperCollins, 2018.

McConnell, Susan. *Somatic Internal Family Systems Therapy: Awareness, Breath, Resonance, Movement, and Touch in Practice.* North Atlantic Books, 2020.

McTaggart, Lynne. *The Field: The Quest for the Secret Force of the Universe.* HarperCollins, 2002.

Melis, Yuri, Emanuela Apicella, Marsia Macario, Eugenia Dozio, Giuseppina Bentivoglio, and Leonardo Mendolicchio. "Trans-Auricular Vagus Nerve Stimulation in the Treatment of Recovered Patients Affected by Eating and Feeding Disorders and Their Comorbidities." *Psychiatria Danubina* 32, Suppl 1 (2020): 42–46. https://pubmed.ncbi.nlm.nih.gov/32890361/.

Motoyama, Hiroshi. *Theories of the Chakras: Bridge to Higher Consciousness.* New Age Books, 1981.

Moyano A., Jairo R., Sara Mejía Torres et al. "Vagus Nerve Neuropathy Related to SARS COV-2 Infection." *IDCases* 26, e01242 (April 2021). https://doi.org/10.1016/j.idcr.2021.e01242.

Mukherjee, Sukhes. "Alcoholism and Its Effects on the Central Nervous System." *Current Neurovascular Research* 10, no. 3 (August 2013): 256–62. https://doi.org/10.2174/15672026113109990004.

"New Evidence Suggests Link Between Gut Health and Parkinson's Disease." Duke Health. Updated December 4, 2023. https://corporate.dukehealth.org/news/new-evidence-suggests-link-between-gut-health-and-parkinsons-disease.

Newton, Michael. *Journey of Souls: Case Studies of Life Between Lives.* 5th ed. Llewellyn Publications, 2009.

Novak, David J., and Maurice Victor. "The Vagus and Sympathetic Nerves in Alcoholic Polyneuropathy." *Archives of Neurology* 30, no. 4 (April 1974): 272–84. doi:10.1001/archneur.1974.00490340001001.

Ober, Clinton, Stephen T. Sinatra, and Martin Zucker. *Earthing: The Most Important Health Discovery Ever!* Basic Health Publications, 2014.

Ogden, Pat, and Janina Fisher. *Sensorimotor Psychotherapy: Interventions for Trauma and Attachment.* W. W. Norton, 2015.

Ogden, Pat, Kekuni Minton, and Clare Pain. *Trauma and the Body: A Sensorimotor Approach to Psychotherapy.* W.W. Norton, 2006.

Oschman, James L., Gaétan Chevalier, and Richard Brown. "The Effects of Grounding (Earthing) on Inflammation, the Immune Response, Wound Healing, and Prevention and Treatment of Chronic Inflammatory and Autoimmune Diseases." *Journal of Inflammation Research* 8 (March 2015): 83–96. https://doi.org/10.2147/JIR.S69656.

Panksepp, Jaak, and Lucy Biven. *The Archaeology of Mind: Neuroevolutionary Origins of Human Emotions.* W.W. Norton, 2012.

Parkman, Henry P. "Idiopathic Gastroparesis." *Gastroenterology Clinics of North America* 44, no. 1 (March 2015): 59–68. https://doi.org/10.1016/j.gtc.2014.11.015.

Pearlman, Laurie Anne, Camille B. Wortman, Catherine A. Feuer, Christine Farber, and Therese A. Rando. *Treating Traumatic Bereavement: A Practitioner's Guide*. Guildford Press, 2014.

Peirce, Penney. *Frequency: The Power of Personal Vibration*. Atria Books/Beyond Words, 2009.

Porges, Stephen W. "The Polyvagal Perspective." *Biological Psychology* 74, no. 2 (February 2007): 116–43. https://doi.org /10.1016%2Fj.biopsycho.2006.06.009.

Porges, Stephen W. *Polyvagal Perspectives: Interventions, Practices, and Strategies*. W. W. Norton, 2024.

Porges, Stephen W. *Polyvagal Safety: Attachment, Communication, Self-Regulation*. W. W. Norton, 2021.

Porges, Stephen W. *The Polyvagal Theory: Neurophysiological Foundations of Emotions, Attachment, Communication, and Self-Regulation*. W. W. Norton, 2011.

Porges, Stephen W. "Vagal Tone: An Autonomic Mediator for Affect." In *The Development of Emotion Regulation and Dysregulation*, edited by Judy Garber and Kenneth A. Dodge. Cambridge University Press, 2010.

Porges, Stephen, and Deb Dana, eds. *Clinical Applications of the Polyvagal Theory: The Emergence of Polyvagal-Informed Therapies*. W. W. Norton, 2018.

Porges, Stephen W., and Stephen Porges. *Our Polyvagal World: How Safety and Trauma Change Us*. W. W. Norton, 2023.

Richo, David. *How to Be an Adult: A Handbook on Psychological and Spiritual Integration*. Paulist Press, 1991.

Robertson, Robin. *Indra's Net: Alchemy and Chaos Theory as Models for Transformation*. Quest Books, 2009.

Rosenberg, Stanley. *Accessing the Healing Power of the Vagus Nerve: Self-Help Exercises for Anxiety, Depression, Trauma, and Autism*. North Atlantic Books, 2017.

Samuels, Andrew, Bani Shorter, and Fred Plaut. "Individuation." In *A Critical Dictionary of Jungian Analysis*. Routledge & Kegan Paul, 1986.

Schwartz, Arielle, *Applied Polyvagal Theory in Yoga: Therapeutic Practices for Emotional Health*. W. W. Norton, 2024.

Schwartz, Arielle, and Barb Maiberger. *EMDR Therapy and Somatic Psychology: Interventions to Enhance Embodiment in Trauma Treatment*. W. W. Norton, 2018.

Schwartz, Richard C., and Martha Sweezy. *Internal Family Systems Therapy*. Guilford Press, 2020.

Schiopu, Cristina, Gabriela Ştefănescu, and Smaranda Diaconescu et al. "Magnesium Orotate and the Microbiome-Gut-Brain Axis Modulation: New Approaches in Psychological Comorbidities of Gastrointestinal Functional Disorders." *Nutrients* 14, no. 8 (April 2022): 1567.

Shaik-Dasthagirisaheb, Yazdani, Giuseppe Varvara, Giovanna Murmura et al. "Role of Vitamins D, E and C in Immunity and Inflammation." *Journal of Biological Regulators and Homeostatic Agents* 27, no. 2 (2013): 291–95.

Shapiro, Francine. *Getting Past Your Past: Take Control of Your Life with Self-Help Techniques from EMDR Therapy*. Rodale Books, 2012.

Shapiro, Francine. *Eye Movement Desensitization and Reprocessing: Basic Principles, Protocols, and Procedures*. Guilford Press, 2001.

Siegel, Daniel J. *The Developing Mind: How Relationships and the Brain Interact to Shape Who We Are*. Guilford Press, 1999.

Shapiro, Francine. *Mindsight: The New Science of Personal Transformation*. Bantam Books, 2010.

Siegel, Daniel J., Allan N. Schore, and Louis Cozolino, eds. *Interpersonal Neurobiology and Clinical Practice*. W. W. Norton, 2021.

Sogyal, Rinpoche. *The Tibetan Book of Living and Dying*. Edited by Patrick Gaffney and Andrew Harvey. HarperCollins, 2002.

Stein, Amy. *Heal Pelvic Pain: The Proven Stretching, Strengthening, and Nutrition Program for Relieving Pain, Incontinence, IBS, and Other Symptoms Without Surgery*. McGraw-Hill, 2008.

Sweezy, Martha. *Internal Family Systems for Shame and Guilt*. Guilford Press, 2023.

Taha, Amira Mohamed, Amr Elrosasy, Ahmed S. Mohamed et al. "Effects of Non-Invasive Vagus Nerve Stimulation on Inflammatory Markers in COVID-19 Patients: A Systematic Review and Meta-Analysis of Randomized Controlled Trials." *Cureus* 16, no. 10: e70613. doi:10.7759/cureus.70613.

Tatkin, Stan. *Wired for Love: How Understanding Your Partner's Brain and Attachment Style Can Help You Defuse Conflict and Build a Secure Relationship*. New Harbinger Publications, 2010.

Van der Kolk, Bessel. *The Body Keeps the Score: Brain, Mind, and Body in the Healing of Trauma*. Penguin Publishing Group, 2015.

"Vasovagal Syncope." Cleveland Clinic. Updated June 19, 2022. www.https//my.clevelandclinic.org/health/symptoms/23325 -vasovagal-syncope.

Vickhoff, Björn, Helge Malmgren, Rickard Åström et al. "Music Structure Determines Heart Rate Variability of Singers." *Frontiers in Psychology* 4, no. 334 (July 2013). doi:10.3389 /fpsyg.2013.00334.

Vieira, C., S. Evangelista, R. Cirillo et al. "Effect of Ricinoleic Acid in Acute and Subchronic Experimental Models of Inflamma- tion." *Mediators of Inflammation* 9, no. 5 (2000): 223–28. https:// doi.org/10.1080/09629350020025737.

Wang, Connie X., Isaac A. Hilburn, Daw-An Wu et al. "Transduc- tion of the Geomagnetic Field as Evidenced from Alpha-Band Activity in the Human Brain." *eNeuro* 6, no. 2 (March 2019): ENEURO.0483-18.2019. https://doi.org/10.1523 /ENEURO.0483-18.2019.

Weiss, Brian. *Many Lives, Many Masters.* Simon & Schuster, 1988.

Weiss, Brian. *Only Love Is Real: A Story of Soulmates Reunited.* Grand Central Publishing, 1997.

Welwood, John. *Toward a Psychology of Awakening: Buddhism, Psy- chotherapy, and the Path of Personal and Spiritual Transformation.* Shambala: 2002.

Wilson, James L. *Adrenal Fatigue: The 21st Century Stress Syndrome.* Smart Publications, 2001.

Yogananda, Paramahansa. *Autobiography of a Yogi.* Crystal Clarity Publishing, 2005.

Zappaterra, Mauro. "Connection to Source via the Cerebrospinal Fluid." https://scienceandnonduality.com/videos/connection -to-source-via-the-cerebrospinal-fluid/.

Zindel, Segal V., J. Mark G. Williams, John D. Teasdale. *Mindfulness-Based Cognitive Therapy for Depression*. Guildford Press, 2018.

Zukav, Gary. *The Seat of the Soul*. Simon & Schuster, 1989.

To Write to the Author

If you wish to contact the author or would like more information about this book, please write to the author in care of Llewellyn Worldwide Ltd. and we will forward your request. Both the author and publisher appreciate hearing from you and learning of your enjoyment of this book and how it has helped you. Llewellyn Worldwide Ltd. cannot guarantee that every letter written to the author can be answered, but all will be forwarded. Please write to:

C. J. Llewelyn
℅ Llewellyn Worldwide
2143 Wooddale Drive
Woodbury, MN 55125-2989
Please enclose a self-addressed stamped envelope for reply,
or $1.00 to cover costs. If outside the U.S.A., enclose
an international postal reply coupon.

Many of Llewellyn's authors have websites with additional information and resources. For more information, please visit our website at http://www.llewellyn.com.